THE
DEADLY
EMOTIONS

THE
DEADLY
EMOTIONS

The Role of Anger, Hostility, and Aggression in Health and Emotional Well-being

Ernest H. Johnson

PRAEGER

New York
Westport, Connecticut
London

Library of Congress Cataloging-in-Publication Data

Johnson, Ernest H.
    The deadly emotions : the role of anger, hostility, and aggression
in health and emotional well-being / Ernest H. Johnson.
      p.   cm.
    Includes bibliographical references and index.
    ISBN 0-275-93590-6
    1. Emotions—Health aspects.   2. Mental health.   I. Title.
  RC455.4.E46J64   1990
   616.07'1—dc20   90-35100

British Library Cataloguing in Publication Data is available.

Library of Congress Catalog Card Number: 90-35100
ISBN: 0-275-93590-6

First published in 1990

Praeger Publishers, One Madison Avenue, New York, NY 10010
An imprint of Greenwood Publishing Group, Inc.

Printed in the United States of America

The paper used in this book complies with the
Permanent Paper Standard issued by the National
Information Standards Organization (Z39.48-1984).

10 9 8 7 6 5 4 3 2 1

For my family:
my mother, Evelyn,
my father, Nathaniel, and my stepfather, Dan;
my sisters, Danette and Karen,
my brothers, Dennis and Arthur

And the New Generation,
Denetria and Brandon

For several mentors, colleagues, and special friends
who allowed me to benefit from their wisdom:
Drs. Charles Spielberger, Ernest Harburg,
Lillian Gleiberman, Stevo Julius, James Jackson,
Ray Rosenman, and W. Doyle Gentry

Contents

Figures and Tables

FIGURES

TABLES

THE
DEADLY
EMOTIONS

Introduction

I would like to start out by describing the circumstances, or, as some say, the major stimulus, that prompted me to write this book. I guess that I took a very deep and critical look at my previous training as a clinical–behavioral psychologist and my current research on the emotional determinants of hypertension after reading the very influential books Anger: The Misunderstood Emotion by Carol Tavris,[1] and "The Dance of Anger," by Harriet Goldhor Lerner[2]. After reading these two books, I was convinced that there was still much to say about the role of emotions in human disease and suffering. However, two years then went by while I was trying to set up the appropriate contingencies—winning a major lottery and becoming a millionaire; cloning myself so that I could double my earnings—that would allow me to write the book that you are reading. Since it took so long to accomplish these relatively "small" setup goals, I thought it best to go ahead and write the book without them. So goes the theory of contingent behaviors!

In the book written by Carol Tavris, she describes the anatomy of anger, and does a great job describing the impact of anger on both psychological and physical well–being. Whereas I strongly agree with Tavris's notion that anger is a misunderstood emotion, I would go even further and make the claim that anger is not only misunderstood, but deadly. Anger erodes our coronary arteries as well as our relationships with loved ones—even those whom we promised to love until death summons us to the promised land. And anger is often accompanied by other emotions such as anxiety, fear, guilt, shame, and depression. Some say that anger is insanity because it is so often accompanied by negative and destructive thoughts. Others believe that the very causes of anger are strongly associated with something about ourselves that is unacceptable to ourselves.

From a historical perspective, the book you are reading invokes the spirit—or if you will permit me—the negative vibes of the times. Just behind us are the ages of anxiety, and then Aquarius, and now an age of cynicism, economic disaster, racial hardships, child and spouse abuse, broken families, and a disbelief in the magic and power of strong family bonds; an age of drunken disobedience and misguided and violent youth gangs; an age of designer jeans and designer drugs; an age of transition into the twenty–first century which expands further than our imagination; an age when people attempt to develop and sustain their individuality by hiding in front of television or tuning to their Walkman radios. All right, then, I do sound a bit cynical. It may be that you have the makings of a good psychologist.

According to the Zeitgeist, I can openly admit and express the feelings of anger and irritability that I have encountered throughout my life. It is supposed to be good for my psychological well–being and my blood pressure for me to admit and express these feelings that I have been "conditioned" to suppress. In my opinion, the real truth of the matter is that we have all become conditioned to mistrust our own emotional and bodily reactions to both painful and pleasurable events. On one hand, we have lost faith in the belief that mankind and womankind can give unconditional love; and on the other hand, we are afraid and angered by the thought of losing the very love that we are afraid to cultivate. We live in a time in which it is highly approved that we seek solitude by running ten miles a day, rather than take a leisurely long walk with family members or close friends. We live in a time of the Great Hidden Agendas, we are constantly looking for the motives behind the behavior of others. In other words, we have become extremely untrusting.

Today thousands of people around the world will begin their day with a moderate workout (perhaps a 5–10-mile jog or run) that starts at 6:00 a.m. and has to be completed by exactly 7:00 a.m. in order to shower, "visit" with the spouse (or partner), dress, eat breakfast, drop the kids off, and arrive at work by 8:00 a.m. There is nothing wrong with this picture—we all want to be healthy, wealthy, and wise! The issue that it raises—in terms of my interests in this book—is the difference in the physiological state of the human body when exercising as compared to when angry and under considerable stress. Believe it or not, there are more similarities than there are differences. So why is it that exercising until our hearts are content and pumped full of adrenaline is all right while being angry and stressed–out is so bad for us? The truth will be unveiled in this book. I have attempted to assemble its information in such a way as to be readable for the general public as well as those friends and colleagues who—like myself—are deeply engaged in studying the role of emotions and personality factors on physical health. I have tried to present a balanced review of a complex topic; and I believe that the book will be of interest to many groups including psychologists, psychiatrists, physiologists, biological scientists, epidemiologists, and students undergoing training in behavioral medicine/health psychology and medicine.

The idea that the mind can influence the body is the foundation of psychosomatic medicine and the relatively new field of inquiry referred to as "behavioral medicine." The effects of anger, hostility, anxiety, and depression on the nervous system and glandular secretions—and eventually on organs, muscles, bone, and blood—are well-known, but not well understood or accepted by all scientists. If all of our emotions are expressed through physiological processes that are the result of complex mechanisms under the influence of the nervous system, then the first danger to health and life may be our emotional well-being, rather than the invading germs.

Although I may be accused of premature speculation—of going beyond the limits of research data currently available—I believe that the research evidence integrated for this book offers sufficient support for the notion that Anger–Hostility–Aggression—The AHA! Syndrome—contributes to poor psychological functioning and may have a deadly role in the pathogenesis of several health problems such as heart disease and cancer that are the cause of death for many people throughout the world. Certainly, new data regarding the relationships between emotions and health are constantly emerging, and the links between emotions and physical health are far from being totally understood. But there is no question that the links exist, and it is about time that all of us (the general public, researchers, physicians, and psychologists) recognize that certain emotions may play a deadly role in human suffering and disease.

Still an important caution is in order. It has to do with the age–old question of direction of causality, or which came first—the chicken or the egg? The simple truth is that both the chicken and the egg exist, and one could develop a multitude of theories about which existed first. In a similar way, the etiological factors that contribute to chronic diseases in mankind run the range from genetic to sociocultural. In my opinion, the causes of most human disease are from multiple factors. The issue is not whether genetic, physiological, social, or psychological factors play a role in the pathogenesis of health problems, but rather how much of the cause can be attributed to psychological and emotional factors or whether psychological factors affect the progression of human disease. But again, there is the question of the causal order of events. Which came first—the emotional and psychological difficulties related to the management of Anger Hostility Aggression, or the health problems? In many cases, "correlations"—or the concurrent relationship—between emotions and health problems are the driving force behind the hypothesis that Anger Hostility Aggression contributes to the development of poor health. Although a number of methodological weaknesses (e.g., observations based on too small a number of subjects; absence of appropriate control groups inaccurate reporting of psychological and health status) may sometimes be identified among the studies reviewed in this book, there is no question that the links between emotions and physical illness exist.

The book is divided into seven major chapters. In Chapter 1, I will describe the association between anger, hostility, and aggression: the AHA! Syndrome. The anatomy of the AHA! Syndrome will be examined along with the question of why we see red. The final part of Chapter 1 looks at the relationship between the AHA! Syndrome and mortality from heart disease, cancer, and all causes combined.

Chapter 2 explores the role of the AHA! Syndrome in health and psychological well–being. The mechanisms, potentially responsible for the relationship between the AHA! Syndrome and health are introduced. I also examine the linkage between suppressed anger and depression. In the final part of Chapter 2, the connection between stress, the fight/flight syndrome, and the AHA! Syndrome are discussed.

In Chapter 3, I will review and discuss the available research describing the relationship between cardiovascular disease and the AHA! Syndrome. Particular attention is given to the various studies on the so–called hypertensive personality and to research describing the lethal role of the AHA! Syndrome in coronary heart disease. The final part of the chapter reviews some of the current research on the relationship between emotions and cholesterol.

Chapter 4 will present current research describing the psychological factors in cancer, ulcers, cigarette smoking, and psoriasis.

Chapter 5 is a review of relevant research literature describing the role of Anger Hostility Aggression in child and spouse abuse. I will discuss research findings which indicate that talking about or talking out anger is not the best way to get it out of your system. The role of family stress and other sources of frustration as triggers of abuse will be discussed, along with the contribution of alcohol consumption to problems of anger and hostility management.

In Chapter 6, I will describe the available research on gender and ethnic differences in the experience and/or expression of anger. We will approach the question pertaining to which sex has the problem with anger. The final part of this chapter discusses whether or not black Americans are more prone to anger than white Americans. The origin of anger–coping styles in black Americans will also be explored.

Chapter 7 investigates some of the psychological treatment approaches for regulating anger and exaggerated emotional responses to stress. Applications of these techniques to the treatment of hypertension and coronary heart disease will be discussed. The final part of the chapter describes a number of general strategies for managing anger.

Each chapter represents an integration of research and clinical findings from a wide range of professionals. I hope to serve as an organizer and interpreter of the research on the relationship between the AHA! Syndrome and both physical and psychological health. I assume full responsibility for the interpretation employed here—an interpretation that has relevance to the field of psychosomatic medicine and the relatively new field referred to as "behavioral medicine." I have attempted to integrate my own research findings into the discussion at various points in this book.

A notes section is provided for each chapter, and I hope that these serve as further reading and study sources for readers' special interests. Finally, I hope that my book will be an inspiration and guide to those in the business of helping people cope with emotional difficulties. And although chapter 7 does explore some of the psychological treatment approaches for dealing with anger and hostility problems, it is not recommended as a presciptive manual. Professional help should be sought if you have concerns about your capability in managing the Anger Hostility Aggression in your life.

1

Anger, Hostility, and Aggression: The AHA! Syndrome

Anger, hostility, and aggression have recently emerged from the black box that contains our worst wishes and thoughts to be considered as potential risk factors for cardiovascular diseases and other health problems. From a historical point of view, the maladaptive effects of these negative emotions in the etiology of psychological difficulties such as depression, neuroses, and schizophrenia have long been emphasized. Anger, particularly when manifested as chronic hostility, has recently been linked with the Type–A behavior pattern, coronary heart disease (CHD), death from CHD and malignant neoplasms, and death from all causes combined. Interestingly enough, a number of studies relate high levels of anger and hostility to the classic risk factors (e.g., cholesterol, smoking, drinking) that have been shown to predict heart disease, cancer, and other major health problems. In addition to these relatively recent attempts to link personality factors to poor physical health, scientists studying more psychosomatic illness over the past 40 years have revealed a rather consistent relationship between essential hypertension (high blood pressure) and problematic styles of expressing anger. Suppressed anger, or the tendency to experience intense feelings of anger but not express them, has also been shown to be related to rheumatoid arthritis and malignant breast cancer in women. Problematic ways of coping with anger and abrasive marital relationships not only erode the love even between couples once so much in love that they were almost inseparable, but also contribute to both child and spouse abuse. As current studies of women and men undergoing marital separation/divorce also show, the degree of psychological distress caused by such an unpleasant proceeding leads to adverse immunological changes that probably increase the incidence of infectious diseases.

Although there are hundreds of articles published in the medical literature discussing the linkage between poor physical health and psychological factors, the majority of physicians simply pay lip service to the idea. One of the reasons for this lack of acceptance has to do with the fact that few studies have looked at the actual mechanisms by which negative emotional states and psychological distress contribute to the onset of the disease. Another reason is that most physicians and biomedical researchers are not well trained in the language of psychology. The reverse is just as true for psychologists: Most are not very familiar with the language of medicine and physiology. Within the past decade there have been major efforts devoted to a kind of "cross–fertilization" between medicine and psychology. This has been accomplished by way of post–doctoral training of psychologists in the language and biomedical measurements associated with medicine. Being myself one of the products of this union, I am hopeful that this book will provide you with fresh insight about the role of emotions in health and well–being. In the case of what I call the "AHA! Syndrome," for example, could it be that angry and hostile individuals tend to engage in poor health practices (i.e., no physical exercise, not wearing seat belts, and eating lousy diets high in cholesterol, and managing to—as my grandma once said,— "smoke like a chimney and drink until they drop")? Or could it be that a deadly biological and physiological deterioration that erodes our coronary arteries and disrupts the immune system is directly related to the experience of intense feelings of anger and hostility?

DEFINITION AND PSYCHOLOGY OF THE AHA! SYNDROME

Take a moment and think about the last time you became angry. Consider a situation where you were so angry and upset that you thought you would explode and lose control—a time when you thought you were on the brink of a nervous breakdown. In fact, take a few moments and respond to the questions in Appendix A. They are presented so that you might have a better idea of the situational determinants of your anger.

"Anger" is generally considered to be an emotional state consisting of feelings of irritation, annoyance, fury, and rage along with heightened activation of the autonomic nervous system and the endocrine system, tension in the skeletal musculature, antagonistic thought patterns, and at the same time aggressive behaviors. This complex emotional–physiological pattern can be more easily elicited in interpersonal and social situations among individuals who are more prone or have a strong trait to experience anger.

In thinking about anger, it is important to distinguish between the experience (frequency, intensity, duration) of anger and the expression of anger, the latter which might be best conceptualized as a transactional response to provocations that serves to regulate the emotional discomforts associated with problematic interpersonal relationships.[1–5] With regards to the expression of anger, three coping styles have been identified in the current research literature: (1) Anger–In, (2) Anger–Out, and (3) Anger–Control/Reflection.[2] The first style—Anger–In—refers to individuals who frequently experience intense angry feelings, but tend to suppress these feelings rather than express them verbally or physically. An excellent example of the suppressed–anger coping style often occurs in the work environment, usually when a supervisor gets angry and blows up at an employee for reasons that appear unimportant to the employee. The usual response of the employee is to become angry and upset, but in most cases the feelings of anger are not openly expressed. The second coping style—Anger–Out—is characterized by the frequent experience of anger that is expressed in aggressive behaviors directed toward other people or objects in the environment. Anger–Out may be expressed in physical acts such as slamming doors, pounding on tabletops or desks, throwing objects, or assaulting other persons. Anger–Out can also be expressed verbally in the form of insults, threats, criticism, sarcasm, or the extreme use of profanity. Finally, the third coping style—Anger–Control/Reflection—is characterized by a concerted attempt to constrain and control angry feelings and solve the problem(s) that are the focus of the provocation.[1] There is a great deal of energy and effort invested in monitoring and preventing the experience and expression of anger.

At first glance, one might assume that the Anger–Control/Reflection coping style is the best way to manage anger. In some circumstances, controlling anger is highly desirable, but the over–control of anger could result in withdrawal, passivity, severe anxiety reactions, strained interpersonal relationships, and depression.

The concept of "hostility" is much broader and usually involves angry feelings, but has the added connotation of negative, destructive attitudes such as hatred, animosity, and resentment. In many instances, hostility motivates aggressive and vindictive behaviors. While it should be clear that anger and hostility both refer to feelings and attitudes, the concept of "aggression "is generally used to describe destructive and punitive behaviors. As you can see, anger is a more elementary concept than hostility or aggression.[2] While neither a necessary nor a sufficient condition for the development of hostile attitudes and the manifestation of aggressive behaviors, anger often leads to hostility and aggression.

There is an extensive body of research—some of which will be reviewed in this book—showing that anger arousal increases the probability of aggression and hostility. Moreover, a considerable proportion of the acts of aggravated assault and homicide involves an angry perpetrator. Many instances of criminal assault are not simply the result of a discrete event, but occur because of an escalating sequence of antagonistic thoughts and behavioral responses. In the case of family or domestic violence—whether between husband and wife, or problems in disciplining a child—the failure to manage anger constructively is typically the cause of the problem. Unfortunately, the concepts of anger, hostility, and aggression—taken together, The AHA! Syndrome—are often used interchangeably in the research literature as well as among the lay public. This has caused anger, which is a normal and fundamental emotion, to acquire a bad reputation stemming from the fact that many people have not learned how to handle their anger properly.

This association of anger with hostility and aggression engenders a belief that anger is negative and harmful, because it is then expected that anger will escalate into aggressive and hostile behaviors or result in some tragic event. The mere fact of becoming angry about something and making this known is enough to put others on the alert that we are out of control, driven by a passion that has taken control of the personality. However, only a small proportion of our angry experiences result in hostility and an overtly aggressive behavioral reaction toward other people. According to psychologist Raymond Novaco, anger becomes problematic when it: (1) occurs too frequently, (2) occurs too intensely, (3) lasts too long, (4) leads to hostile attitudes and aggressive behavioral responses, (5) disrupts family and work relationships, and (6) has a bad effect on one's health. For the most part, there has been inadequate attention paid to the experience or expression of anger as a style of coping with stressful life problems.[6]

The words "anger", "hostility", and "aggression" evoke images of violent mobs rioting through the streets, frustrated motorists erupting in fist fights, and enraged spouses and lovers slamming doors and throwing objects at each other. Anger expressed the wrong way—as aggressiveness—can lead to the kind of violence that now seems to permeate our society. On the other hand, unexpressed and over-controlled anger can linger on consciously and may cripple people emotionally—leaving them depressed, anxious, and probably a bit confused about their state of emotional well–being. In many instances, intense and prolonged feelings of anger lead to the individual's not being able to think straight and clearly focus on the nature of the provocation. Individuals experiencing intense rage probably also experience a major break down in their perceptions of reality as well as in the accuracy of their judgments in troubled interpersonal relationships: They just do not know what is really going on around them.

Anger is by no means a reflexive, automatic response to provoking events. Cognitive factors such as one's future expectations and appraisals are often centrally involved in the experience, expression, and degree of control of anger, as well as its maintenance and dissipation. Anger can either subside rapidly or else be repressed; and as indicated earlier, anger can be the stimulus for a wide range of emotions such as anxiety, depression, and guilt. If repression takes place as a defensive mechanism in managing anger, the anger response becomes excluded from awareness. The anger may then reemerge into consciousness when events are experienced that are associated with the original repression of the event responsible for the provocation.

To illustrate the point we may examine a problem that is common to many newlywed couples and a major source of marital dissatisfaction— not having enough money. In this example, Mark and Amy have been married for about two years. Mark is employed full–time as a medical technician and Amy works as a secretary. Their combined yearly take home salary is $28,000. This may sound like a nice sum, but—with house and insurance payments that total to $1,000, two car payments and insurance that come to $700 ($350 for each car), the usual monthly expenses (electricity, gas, water, heating, phone) amounting to $250, and medical and life insurance of $200—this couple does not have much money for food or fun on the $2300 a month they bring home. They are even falling behind in the payment of several monthly bills. And in fact, their lack of money has been the source of many arguments and fights. They blame each other for the difficulties, and the situation has gotten to the point that they are always upset and angry at each other. For the most part, the feelings of anger, irritability, and dissatisfaction about their relationship are really centered around their financial difficulties. Let us suppose that Mark has attempted to cope with his money anxiety by repressing the feeling and excluding it from awareness. This sounds all well and good, except that Mark has started to become intensely enraged when funds get tight near the end of the month. Moreover, Mark's anger gets out of control, and he is even further enraged when he has to bring a lunch from home. The very act of preparing the lunch reminds him just how angry and upset he is about the financial situation. Not only does Mark feel angry about having to bring a lunch from home; also he feels ashamed, embarrassed, and to a certain degree guilty and resentful about his inability to resolve the problem. The situation is made worse when Mark starts to drink heavily. Now he not only blames Amy for the financial problems, but also accuses her of being the reason for his drinking and their marital difficulties. Had Mark not repressed his anger, it is quite possible that the difficulties he and Amy are experiencing would not be so severe.

Another phenomenon often associated with anger—and partly the blame for the bad reputation that anger has received—is referred to as "displaced anger." When circumstances prevent an individual from expressing anger toward an offending stimulus (whether person, object, or situation), he or she may direct that anger toward someone or something else. The classic example is the husband who arrives home from a bad day at the office and immediately yells at the kids or proceeds to insult his wife by telling her how awful dinner was the previous evening or how bad the house looks. Displacement is a common emotional process, and appears with particular frequency in dreams. Usually, the anger response itself corresponds to the dreamer's real attitude. In some dreams, however, the response is not anger, but just the opposite. Although there are times when the content of the dream may be identical to the awake–state stimulus and anger response, Sigmund Freud emphasized that there is more often a displacement of emotional reactions in dreams.

In any event, there is probably a great deal of individuality in the rate of acceleration and deceleration of the anger response. In some people, feelings of anger and irritability pass rapidly; in others, they linger consciously and in dreams for a considerable period of time. But as indicated earlier, anger can be a highly constructive tool. It serves to alert us that something is wrong and provides the impetus to make changes. The key to the healthy management of anger is not only to express it, but to express it appropriately—in ways that focus on the events and circumstances that triggered the anger in the first place.

THE ANATOMY OF THE AHA! SYNDROME

In order to understand the nature of the AHA! syndrome, we found it useful to develop a basic model that would explain why most individuals experience that basic and misunderstood emotional response called "anger". I say "we" because the model emerged from research with colleagues at the University of Michigan (psychologist Ernest Harburg) and the University of South Florida (psychologist Charles D. Spielberger). The model is quite simple: Anger is conceptualized as a psychophysiologic response (involving negative feeling states, antagonistic thoughts, and heightened physiological activation) that is induced by social situations wherein the individual perceives (1) a loss or threat of loss of (2) something felt to be possessed (rights, job, marriage, or physical objects), through (3) perceived arbitrary and unfair and unjustifiable acts by others (person, group, or society). When the loss is sudden, is perceived to be highly arbitrary, and involves a matter strongly valued by the individual, then the feelings of anger and irritability will be intensely experienced. The intensity and duration of the anger episode will likely be prolonged if the time it would take to change the situation is perceived as being too long. The fact that frustration is a frequent component of the anger response is clearly demonstrated in the "waiting situation," in which sensitivity to the duration will result in irritation, uneasiness, discomfort, dissatisfaction, tension, sighing, and frequent rhythmic movement of the hands and feet.

One of several coping responses to provocation is suppressed anger. If this response is consistently and chronically evoked across many social situations, then a state of hostility and resentment will most assuredly arise. In this state, psychophysiological processes are aroused by the internal attitude. The blood pressure and heart rate increase, muscles remain tensed and so on. In other words, anger that is chronically experienced and that erodes into bitter resentment and hostility stimulates the so-called fight or flight response. The heart pumps dramatically to increase blood pressure and provide blood to the muscles necessary for action. At the same time, blood vessels constrict in the skin to minimize bleeding. A flood of hormones—mostly noradrenaline and cortisol—is released to drive and buffer the body's resources.

As I shall illustrate later in this book, the psychophysiological responses associated with the experience of anger can be destructive over the long term, and may be viewed as specific stressors that disrupts the body's biochemical balance and the workings of its immune system. The hormones released by anger and sustained by maladaptive ways of coping with anger—if not used up in some way—may deposit in the walls of constricted blood vessels, perhaps contributing to the development of atherosclerotic plagues and the eventual development of coronary heart disease. This disruption of the body's biochemical balance that is related to the AHA! Syndrome may also be associated with other varying health consequences such as tumor growth, lung and breast cancer, and substance abuse (e.g., alcohol, cigarettes).

Although reviews of the literature on theories of anger, hostility, and aggression reflect a great deal of conceptual ambiguity and confusion, the images evoked by these three words are consistently quite violent. This is interesting in view of the fact that the terms have been defined in different ways by different theorists. But, in my opinion, anger is the core element of both hostility and aggression. Etymologically, the English word "anger" is derived from the old Norse word angre, which means affliction (Latin ad and fligere to strike toward). In Spanish enojar "to get angry" derives from en and ojo something that offends the eye; the noun enojo also signifies disgust. Another Spanish term for anger is enfado trouble. In German, anger is the noun of ang. which means wicked. Anger is the emotional response to wicked stimuli. In French, something chagrin (from the old French graignier) translates into anger. In psychology, etymology is often a useful aid. All these languages, for instance, depict anger as a response to an offending stimulus that elicits resentment, uneasiness, and displeasure.

For the most part, anger has been conceptualized as an emotional state by most theorists and researchers, although different aspects of this emotion are emphasized in the various definitions. For example, psychologists Raymond Novaco and Stanley Schachter define anger in terms of both physiological and cognitive variables[6,7], whereas K.F. Moyer defines it exclusively in terms of physiological events[8]. For Arnold Buss anger is an emotional response with facial–skeletal and autonomic components[9], whereas Seymour Feshbach sees it as a "mediating affective response" with expressive components[10]. H. Kaufman includes intentionality as well as psychophysiological reactions in his definition of anger, which is "an emotion that involves a physiological arousal state coexisting with fantasized or intended acts culminating in harmful effects on another person."[11]

While there is a great deal of confusion about the definition of anger, it is generally agreed that frustration is a major antecedent or stimulus condition. But what is frustration? What does it mean when people say they "feel frustrated"? In the English language, "frustrate" is a verb meaning to disappoint, and deceive, cause to have no effect, bring to nothing, counteract, nullify, and prevent from achieving an objective.

The psychological meaning of frustration pertains to being prevented from gratifying certain impulses or desires, either conscious or unconscious. Although it is generally agreed that frustration is a major antecedent condition that arouses anger, the term has been used in so many different ways by different theorists to the point that the word "frustration" no longer has a specific meaning. In fact, the ambiguity of the term has caused many modern–day theorists to conclude that frustration is an important but seldom sufficient condition for experiencing anger.

Be that as it may, some psychologists such as Charles Spielberger conceptualize anger as a psychological construct whose manifestations must be differentiated: It can be a transitory emotional state or a relatively stable personality trait.[5,12] Emotional states exist at a given moment in time and at a particular level of intensity—as when you have waited in line for a long time to purchase a ticket to some event, but the person in front of you allows another person to enter the line and they receive the last available ticket. Whereas emotional states are often transitory, they can reoccur when evoked by appropriate stimuli. On the other hand, personality traits reflect individual differences in the tendency to react or behave in a specified manner with predictable regularity over a wide range of situations. Spielberger characterizes "state anger" as a transitory emotional state that may fluctuate in intensity and duration over time.[2] The angry reaction is characterized by feelings of annoyance, irritation, and hate as well as heightened autonomic nervous system activation. Whereas the level of state anger should be high when the individual encounters circumstances that are frustrating, persons who are high in what Spielberger refers to as "trait anger" tend to perceive a larger number of situations as frustrating than persons who are low in Trait Anger. In this context, then trait anger refers to relatively stable individual differences in the tendency to experience anger states, and persons high in trait anger tend to respond frequently to frustrating situations with anger–state elevations of a greater intensity.[5,12]

The hostility component of the AHA! Syndrome refers to an attitudinal tendency to evaluate situations and events as anger provoking. The term "hostility" has been defined by Kaufman and David Buss as an attitude that involves disliking others and evaluating them negatively[11,9], while Berkowitz and Moyer equate the term with aggression—which focuses the attention on behaviors, rather than thoughts and attitudes.[8,13,14] The word "hostility" is derived from the Latin hostis, which means enemy. Enmity is open antagonism against one or many individuals. It is also possible to have hostility against ideas or dogmas, but only when they are represented by persons. Hostility is generally a longlasting affective phenomenon, which—once established—may persist without repeated stimulation. This is one essential difference between hostility and anger. Another difference is that hostility is always directed against a person or persons.

The term "aggression" has also generated a great deal of

confusion in the research literature. While there is general agreement that aggressive behavior involves injury to another organism, the notion of intent dramatically alters the meaning of aggression. For example, including the notion of intent in the definition of aggression assumes that aggression serves only the purpose of inflicting injury. However, it is possible to find aggression that is instrumental and focused on the removal of obstacles between the aggressor and a goal; in which case, injury to another organism may result only incidentally.

As you can see from the discussion above, we psychologists have had an extremely difficult time conceptualizing and defining the concepts of anger, hostility, and aggression. In some respects, it is surprising that the research arenas hosting the discussions and debates over these constructs did not burn down to the ground from all the intellectual heat generated. Given the significant overlap in the conceptual definitions of anger, hostility, and aggression, and the variety of operational procedures used to measure them empirically, my colleagues and I began referring to them collectively as the AHA! Syndrome. The individual who spearheaded this movement was my mentor and close friend Charles D. Spielberger.[12] So there you have it a brief historical sketch of the anatomy of the AHA! Syndrome.

In the next section we will consider the various reasons *why* people become angry. If you are interested in learning about your own anger temperament, then complete the questionnaires in Appendix B.

WHY DO WE "SEE RED"?

Our theorizing about the nature of the AHA! Syndrome has been greatly influenced by the work of Sigmund Freud.[15] In the early writing of Freud, aggression was regarded as a reaction to the thwarting of either pleasure–seeking or pain–avoiding responses. However, throughout his writings Freud gave progressively more attention and importance to aggression as being a destructive and violent side of basic human functioning. By 1927, the events of World War I had transformed his conceptualization of aggression into an elaborate theory about the "death instinct." Within this framework, aggression is viewed as a major instinct that motivates man (and woman) to destroy himself. This self–destructiveness is inhibited by the life instinct, however, which turns the destructive energy away from the self and toward the outer world, and in this way provides an outlet for the forces of the death instinct. Human beings are thus regarded as being caught or entrapped in a conflict between life and death, love and hatred, sex and domination. Moreover, whenever the aggressive drives are not vented against external objects, they are turned back into the self and the unconscious. This inward direction of aggression was considered by Freud to be unhealthy and to underlie the pathogenic process that leads to neuroses and psychoses.

Over the years, Freud's psychodynamic disciples have evolved varying views of his conceptualization of aggression. Some contemporary theorists (e.g., Melanie Klein,[16] H. Nunberg,[17] R. Waelder[18]) have fully accepted Freud's notion of a death instinct, while others (H. Hartmann,[19] A. Storr[20]) have proposed instead the existence of a separate aggressive instinct. Still a third group of theorists (Erich Fromm,[21] Karen Horney,[22] L.J. Saul[23]) decided it is best to dispense with the notion of aggression as an instinct and view it as a purely reactive phenomenon. Interestingly enough, neither Freud nor his contemporaries did much theorizing about anger. If they wrote about anger at all, it was either used interchangeably with aggression or viewed as a less intense expression of aggressive instincts.

Soon after Freud formulated his theory of the death instinct, a group of scientists referred to as "drive theorists" rejected the instinctual model and proposed instead a drive state that motivates aggressive behaviors. The drive theorists were more or less directed by J. Dollard, L.W. Doob, N.E. Miller, O.H. Mowrer, and R.R. Sears.[24] Although their view leans heavily on the early pleasure/pain writings of Freud,[25,26] their theory was stated in behavioral terms within a stimulus—response framework. However, the model made no reference to any emotional state such as anger that would intervene between the frustrating event and the aggressive act. This neglect of emotional reactions has been criticized by several scientists, the most notable being L. Berkowitz[27] and J.S. Brown and II.E. Farber.[28] To fill this gap, Berkowitz focused on anger as an emotional state intervening between frustration and aggression; its intensity was seen as a function of certain aspects of frustration.

Perhaps the issue that has generated the most research and interest within the frustration—aggression literature is the "catharsis hypothesis," which emerged from the hydraulic model. The model postulates that, after its arousal, aggressive energy remains active as a motivating force until discharged by some form of aggressive behavior. The expression of aggression is called "catharsis," and the diminished tendency to aggress as a consequence of such expression is called the "cathartic effect." Furthermore, the hypothesis predicts that, if aggression is not expressed, it may lead to an explosive aggressive discharge or some psychosomatic manifestation such as migraines, ulcers, or hypertension. Catharis was used by Freud and his colleague Josef Breuer to explain why, if we are indeed driven by aggressive instincts, relatively few individuals are acting on these aggressive and violent instincts on any given day.[25]

Jack Hokanson and his colleagues in Florida have put a great deal of effort into studying the catharsis hypothesis in laboratory experiments.[29,30] Results from their studies show that, when given the opportunity to aggress physically or verbally against their antagonist, subjects angered by frustrating events often achieve faster decreases in blood pressure and heart rate than if they are given no opportunity to vent their anger. Although others have corroborated these findings, the cathartic effect could not be elicited when the aggression was expressed in fantasy, if the target of the aggression was unrelated to the source of frustration, or if the counter–aggression was directed toward a frustrator of a higher status than the angered person.[31,32]

Personality factors such as high levels of guilt and anxiety have also been found to moderate counter–aggression. In other words, individuals with high levels of guilt and anxiety about openly displaying an aggressive reaction against the target of anger manifest higher levels of blood pressure following the provocation. Moreover, subsequent studies by Hokanson's team indicate that the physical tension reduction effect of the catharsis phenomenon may not be specific to aggression.[30] More recently, Larry Van Egeren and his associates at Michigan State University have studied the interpersonal determinants of cardiovascular reactivity.[33] The subjects in this study interacted individually with a confederate—a trained research assistant—on a computer–controlled game while their blood pressure, heart rate, and other physiologic measures were being monitored. Prior to the start of the computer game, half the subjects were harassed by the confederate while they attempted to come up with solutions to a difficult cognitive task. The confederate tried to distract these subject from solving the task by talking with them and making rude comments about the types of people who participate in psychological experiments. As you might expect, the results from this study showed that harassed subjects experienced and expressed more irritability and anger, and manifested greater arousal on all of the physiological measures.

So then, why do we "see red"? To repeat our earlier formulation, anger is considered to be a complex psychophysiological response that is induced by social situations wherein the individual perceives and appraises the situation as representing (1) a loss or threat of loss of (2) something felt to be possessed (e.g., rights, job, marriage, or physical objects), through (3) perceived arbitrary and unjustifiable acts by others (e.g., persons, groups, or society). Especially if this loss is felt to be sudden and is perceived to be highly arbitrary—involving a matter strongly valued by the individual—then anger will be experienced.

Among the more contemporary theorists, Magda Arnold is perhaps the first to assign a central role to appraisal in emotional reactions.[34] Arnold maintains that anything we encounter is immediately, automatically, and almost involuntarily appraised. In her scheme of things, any event or situation that is appraised as "good" will be approached, while "bad" things are avoided and "indifferent" events and circumstances are simply ignored. Appraisal is regarded as a complement to perception and it produces a tendency to do something. When this tendency is strong, we call it emotion.

According to Arnold, memory forms the basis of our appraisal processes. Any new events, circumstances, or problems are evaluated in terms of past experiences. New situations also evoke a memory of the affect that we associate with the previous experience. These affective memories relive the past appraisals, and are regarded by Arnold as continually distorting judgment. Arnold maintains that the final phase in the appraisal process is related to imagination: The situation itself plus any relevant affective memories lead us to guess and imagine whether what may happen will be good or bad for us. Therefore, thought processes about angry episodes are dependent on memories of previous angry episodes. Given our past experiences, we devise a plan of action that involves various possibilities for coping with the provocation. In this scheme of things, then, the appraisal that arouses an emotion such as anger, is not abstract: It is instantaneous, deliberate, and highly dependent on the memory of similar events. To a certain extent, the emotional response is based on "intuition."

Another contemporary—Richard Lazarus—concurs with Arnold that appraisal is the central cognitive component in an emotional reaction such as anger.[35,36] However, he disagrees with Arnold on the instantaneous, nonabstract, and intuitive aspects of cognitive appraisal. Lazarus maintains that individuals vary in their disposition toward attending and responding to the stimulus of any event, and that these various dispositions shape our interactions with the environment. It is also hypothesized that our cognitive appraisal of the stimulus event largely determines the emotional response: As our thought appraisals alter, our emotional reactions also change. Lazarus argues that, among all the constantly changing stimuli, we always cope with threat or harm via direct action. Since the success or failure of one direct action or another constantly fluctuates, our thoughts, and hence our emotional reactions also fluctuate. Lazarus postulates two kinds of appraisal processes: (1) primary appraisal, which deals with the issue of threat or nonthreat; and (2) secondary appraisal, which has to do with alternative ways of coping with the threat. According to Lazarus, any stimulus event primarily appraised as threatening will be subjected to a secondary appraisal process. If the secondary appraisal process seeks direct action to remove the threat, then the emotion is defined according to what kind of direct action is taken. We label our emotional reactions as representing anger when we choose to attack, whereas avoidance signifies fear and so on.

The social situations that can provoke anger responses are countless, and most are known to all of us. A few immediately recognizable examples include:

1.   driving—a gentle, quiet drive through the streets of New York, say (a taste of manic Monday or the gridlock), or what about that un-eventful drive home from work a few days ago when someone suddenly cut in front of you, or maybe the driver in front of you suddenly decided to change lanes without signaling;

2.   crowds—long lines everywhere, or that person who let someone
        else into the line ahead of you and they got the last ticket;

3.   noise—such as that from the neighbor's late–night parties, or from
        that new appendage extending from your teenager's ear (you
        know: the"boom box");

4.   time pressures—working with unmanageable and unexpected
        deadlines; and

5.   unfair criticisms—as when you are blamed for something you did
        not do, or for a poorly completed team effort.

Another situation that often occurs at work involves working with
individuals who are highly skilled at making sure that they get the credit
for good work, but who cannot be found when there is a foul–up.

Recently, it has been acknowledged that the female cycle just
before and during menstruation increases the predisposition to
experience anger. While this is by no means a situation common to all
women, it may be said that an increase in the frequency and intensity of
anger responses is likely to occur among women who suffer from
premenstrual tension. Similarly, many individuals are more easily angered
when they are hungry and/or physically exhausted or when there has
been some change in a usually stable situation such as sleeping habits.

It is quite tempting to view human transactions in simple cause–
and–effect terms. In today's world, we so easily blame others for our
feelings of anger, particularly when we feel guilty and ashamed about the
way we behaved when angry. On the other hand, if we are the recipient
of someone else's angry reaction, that person believes that we are
unquestionably the cause of the problem. However, human relationships
do not work well under these circumstances. As discussed later, we can
begin to regard our anger as an indicator that change is needed when we
are capable of sharing our feelings and thoughts without blaming the
other person for them. In order to use anger constructively as a vehicle
for change, it is also important for us not to blame ourselves for the angry
feelings and thoughts that other people have in response to our
behavior. Ultimately, no matter how much we may like to blame others, we
are the only source of our own feelings, thoughts, and behavior.

To illustrate this point, we turn our attention to the following crisis
situation. James and Tina have lived together for several years and raised
a purebred Siamese cat who is a much loved member of their
relationship. Early one morning the cat wakes them up and is very sick.
James thinks the situation demands an immediate visit to the veterinarian.
Tina, on the other hand, does not think that the situation is serious
enough to warrant a visit to the vet, and insists that they wait until the end
of the day. Tina essentially accuses James of overreacting and being too
"childlike and immature" regarding his concerns about the sick cat.

When they arrive home from work at the end of the day, the condition of the cat has worsened. The veterinarian's examination reveals that the cat is indeed seriously ill. He tells James and Tina that their cat "could have died" and that they should have brought her earlier. Armed with this information, James becomes extremely angry and furious at Tina and says that she would have been responsible if anything had happened and that the problem with the cat is all her fault.

What are your thoughts about this situation? Who is responsible for James's anger?

Although it is quite easy to empathize with James because of the outcome, the truth of the matter is that he is blaming Tina for his emotional reactions. Tina is no more responsible for his reactions than she is for the cat getting sick. If we analyze the situation in greater detail, we see that it was Tina's responsibility to clarify her beliefs and take action in accordance with them. In all honesty, she did this; it was her opinion and belief that the cat did not need immediate medical attention and that it would be better to wait until the end of the day to make a decision about visiting the veterinarian. As to James, he is the sole source responsible for clarifying his own thoughts and beliefs about the situation. In this example, James did not do a good job in clarifying his position on the problem. He was obviously quite worried and concerned that the cat needed immediate attention, and, yet he did not take her to the veterinarian. In effect, he too decided to postpone it until after work.

I am in no way suggesting here that James has no right to feel angry at Tina, because he is angry. The reasons for his feelings of anger depend on the immediacy of the problem at hand, his appraisal of the situation, the memory of previous events where there were disagreements with Tina, and probably, a number of other circumstances unique to their relationship. In any case, James is angry and quite disturbed that Tina minimized his fears and concerns, disqualified his perception and thoughts and acted like a know–it–all. No matter how much we sympathize with James's situation though, his anger is his problem. This is not to say that he is wrong or misguided, but it is James and not Tina who has the ultimate responsibility for his feelings and what he decides to do or not to do. It would be wonderful if every experience of anger in our interpersonal relationships were clear–cut and well focused. Unfortunately, in our encounters with anger–provoking situations, we think about previous situations and we use the memory of these situations to help justify our anger and the actions we take. In the example of James and Tina, it is possible even that Tina's response was based on there having been previous occasions when they did immediately take the cat to the vet only to discover that nothing was wrong. Perhaps Tina is responding in such a way as to minimize her anger and irritation about the situation. She may have a fiery temper and is behaving this way to control her temper.

It seems an almost impossible undertaking to convince most people that there is nothing innately associated with these kinds of situations that must inevitably provoke feelings of anger and rage. We all have stories that could be used convincingly to support the notion that anger is an innate characteristic of some people when they encounter provocation. As with most personality and psychological characteristics, there are numerous individual differences as well as general similarities in temperament among people; there are large differences within the similarities of racial groups and even among siblings within the same family. Psychologists Arnold Buss and Robert Plomin believe that there are at least four temperaments that have a strong hereditary component and are therefore stable dimensions of personality: (1) emotionality or intensity of reaction, which appears as "a strong temper, a tendency toward violent mood swings"; (2) sociability, a strong desire to be with others; (3) level of activity, or total energy output; and (4) impulsivity, the tendency to respond to events.[37]

To provide supportive evidence that genetic factors contribute to these personality traits, test scores are usually compared among individuals who share the same genetic makeup. There are also a precious few studies showing similarities in temperament and other factors among identical twins who were separated at birth and had no contact with each other until they were reunited during adulthood. In most cases, the scores of identical twins are more similar than the scores of fraternal twins who share the same environment but do not have the same genetic makeup. A recent study by Timothy Smith and his colleagues at the Department of Psychology of the University of Utah is a great example of the studies being conducted in this area.[38] They examined the correlation of hostility scores derived from the Cook and Medley Hostility Scale, within 60 pair of monozygotic (MZ) and 60 pair of dizygotic (DZ) adult twin pairs whose average age was 38. The results indicated that the correlation between scores for the MZ twin pairs was .47, while for the DZ twins it was .15. The larger correlation for the MZ twins indicated that genetic factors are in part responsible for the similarity in hostility scores of identical (MZ) twins. However, please note that the correlation between hostility scores for the MZ twins was not perfect. This suggest that environmental factors are very much involved in the etiology of hostility.

Although the etiology of chronic anger, hostility, or aggression is largely unknown, many chronically angry and hostile individuals attribute their current attitude and emotional state to previously stressful events such as sibling rivalry, frustrated aspirations, occupational disappointments, and various other reasons. For many of these individuals, role models—especially parents and older siblings—are probably extremely influential in the development of hostile attitudes and abrasive ways of coping with frustrations as in the case of the son who imitates and adopts the angry and hostile coping style of a physically and emotionally abusive father. On the other hand, such early role modeling of the behavior of the parents cannot be regarded as the exclusive cause of chronic difficulties with the AHA! Syndrome, because not all angry and hostile individuals come from homes where the parents had difficulties managing anger and hostility. Undoubtedly, there are a host of other factors involved in the process of provoking anger and other elements of the AHA! Syndrome. For example, some of the most recent evidence concerning the role of parental influences in the development of chronic anger—hostility in children comes from research conducted by Karen Mathews and her colleagues at the University of Pittsburgh.[40] In these studies, it has been found that children with the highest levels of anger and hostility are members of families characterized by a lower level of expressed emotions and less cohesiveness and family support. Other findings show that parents of the Type–A children make less frequent positive remarks and more negative or critical remarks and use more physical and restrictive disciplinary techniques than parents of Type–B children.

Given the methodological limitations of this study, it cannot be concluded that the cause of chronic anger—hostility or Type–A behavior is the family environment. But the findings do suggest that angry and hostile children may be well represented in families where there is less approval for expressing emotions and less cohesiveness among the family members. Perhaps children in these families do not learn effective ways of managing anger because of the high degree of negative/critical remarks, strong disapproval for openly expressing emotions, and the presence of physical and restrictive disciplinary styles.

But still, there is the question, "Why do we see red?" Is it due to the nature of certain social situations in themselves or to innate and genetic factors that we are born with? The answer is probably a little of both. All behavior is inevitably the result of both components, and in all probability, the phenotype of anger is under the effect of a genetic potentiality and an environmental specificity. Unfortunately, the answer to whether the genetic or the environmental factors are more important in anger responses must await future research, which needs to be more complex and thorough than the studies conducted in the past. For example, one of the major difficulties we psychologists must overcome in addressing questions about the nature of anger or any other inherited personality predisposition is to develop better questionnaires and observational procedures that enable us to measure accurately what we think is being measured. We are also confronted with the fact that emotionality and temperament are not static traits but are forever being influenced by the range of our experiences, which are constantly changing. Therefore, one would assume that the anger and rage reactions exhibited by an infant or young child would be uniquely different from that of a college student who received a lower class grade than expected or the professional who lives in Los Angeles and is frequently stuck in rush–hour traffic, or the middle–aged man going through a divorce.

For one thing, the fact that frustration is a frequent component of the anger response clearly suggests that, at the very least, the anger–

causing stimuli would change from infancy to adulthood. For example, in the infant, anger is the most common emotional reaction to stimuli that frustrate such as when someone is putting on their clothes when all they want to do is play or taking toys away from them. As the child continues to grow and develop, the energy associated with angry outbursts is directed toward serviceable ends or the attainment of some object. There comes a time in the development sequence where the frequency of anger reaches a crescendo—when the child knows where and how to use anger to correct a situation. There is also a change in the stimuli that trigger anger as the child enters adolescence. In my opinion, the stimuli become more social in nature—teasing, unfairness, sarcasm, failing in accomplishments. Most parents would agree that the duration of anger episodes become longer when the child reaches adolescence, and that the major stimuli that elicit anger are restraints on desires, thwarting of self–assertion, unwelcome advice, unjust accusations, and interruptions of activities. Unfortunately, his or her parents are perceived as being the motivating force behind much of the adolescent feelings of anger. After that point—after late adolescence—there seems to be not much of a change in the anger–provoking stimuli; much of the red we see as adults is evoked by the thwarting of activities or intentions, and by assaults on our self–esteem and self–worth.

Although there may be differences in the specific circumstances that elicit anger from infancy to adulthood, frustration appears to be the common thread. As far as the behavioral and physiological reactions are concerned, the unfortunate truth is that the psychobiology and biochemistry of the experience of anger is probably similar throughout life, with the major difference (we would hope) being the behavioral reactions exhibited at the time of provocation. Most college students and young adults do not hurl themselves around on the floor while yelling, screaming, and pounding their fists when they are angry and irritated.

As discussed above, the reasons for our angry and hostile reactions are numerous. While efforts to demonstrate the consistency of emotionality and temperament from infancy through childhood to adulthood have often revealed contradictory and inconclusive evidence, there is a growing body of research showing that Anger—Hostility—Aggression have adverse health consequences throughout our development and may be a predictor of early death.

IS SEEING RED BETTER THAN BEING DEAD?

The answer to whether seeing red is better than being dead must be a qualified yes, but seeing too much red is deadly! As indicated earlier, the association between the AHA! Syndrome and health status has long been emphasized by researchers, with particular attention given to cardiovascular disorders such as coronary heart disease and essential hypertension as well as complications due to hypertension. Recently, several well conducted studies have also indicated that the AHA! Syndrome may be the most important "coronary prone behavior" underlying the relationship between the Type–A behavior pattern and both the incidence of coronary heart disease in long–term prospective studies and the severity of basic coronary arteriosclerosis.[41] However, before examining in Chapter 2 the impact of the AHA! Syndrome on specific health problems and health behaviors I have some findings to share with you from studies that have examined the bottom line, or—as other folks call it—the end of the line. In other words, we will look at whether the AHA! Syndrome predicts death.

The overlap of psychology and medicine that is variously referred to as "behavioral medicine" or "health psychology" received its initial encouragement from research on the Type–A, or coronary–prone, behavior pattern described by cardiologist Ray Rosenman and his associate Meyer Friedman.[42] It was recognition of the Type–A behavioral pattern—with its behavioral attributes of time urgency, competitiveness, achievement–striving, and hostility—that brought substance to the notion that the AHA! Syndrome has adverse health consequences. Although several prospective studies in the United States and other countries have related self–attributions of certain components of the AHA! Syndrome to ischemic heart disease, the present discussion will focus on studies that have related the AHA! Syndrome to mortality from all causes combined or to death due specifically to cardiovascular disease.

Diagnostic Coronary Angiography Studies and MMPI Hostility

The medical studies on the relationship between the AHA! Syndrome and cardiovascular disease began with an effort to determine whether Type–A patients undergoing diagnostic coronary angiography would have more severe coronary atherosclerosis than Type–B patients.The diagnostic coronary angiography procedure is conducted to determine the severity of coronary artery disease among patients diagnosed with coronary heart disease as well as the extent of clinically significant stenosis of the coronary arteries among individuals suspected of having coronary heart disease. The results from one of the first studies,[43] conducted at Duke University Medical Center, showed that more than 90 percent of patients with severe coronary artery disease were judged to be Type–A using the structured interview developed by Rosenman and Friedman. To a certain extent, these findings have been replicated by other research investigators in other medical centers.[44–46] However, one of the most alarming findings is the report of a prospective relationship between hostility and risk of coronary heart disease.

The research team at Duke was fortunate in discovering that a hostility measure could be derived from the MMPI (Minnesota Multiphasic

Personality Inventory), a psychological test used previously in studies of initially healthy men whose health status was then followed for periods as long as 25 years after completion of the MMPI. In addition to showing hostility (as derived from the MMPI) to be associated with the degree of coronary artery disease, researchers were then able to relate hostility with subsequent morbidity and mortality. For example, John Barefoot, Grant Dahstrom, and Redford Williams carried out a follow–up study of 255 male physicians who completed the MMPI while in medical school 25 years earlier, when their average age was 25 years.[47] The incidence (9–12 percent) of CHD was substantially greater among men with high hostility scores than the incidence (1.5–3 percent) among men with low hostility scores. As Figure 1–1 shows over the 25–year follow–up period only 2.2 percent of the 136 men with low hostility scores (scores below

Figure 1-1
Twenty–five–year survival in 255 medical students/physicians with low and high hostility scores on MMPI

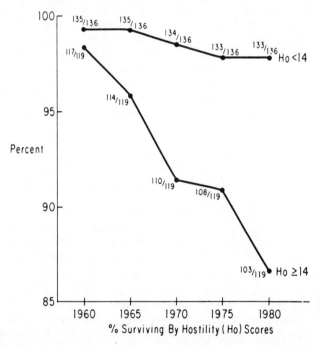

Source: Reprinted with permission from Williams, R. B., Barefoot, J . C., and Shekelle, R. B. The health consequences of hostility, in Chesney, M.A. and Rosenman, R. H. (eds.), Anger and Hostility in Cardiovascular and Behavioral Disorders, p. 179. Washington, D. C.: Hemisphere Publishing/ McGraw–Hill, 1985.

the median of 14) died, while 13.4 percent of the 119 physicians with high hostility scores died. In other words, the incidence of angina pectoris, myocardial infarction, and death from coronary heart disease was discovered to be nearly five times greater among individuals with high MMPI hostility scores than among individuals with low hostility scores. High hostility scores were found to be predictive of death from all causes combined as well as from coronary heart disease.

In a similar study of 1,877 men in the Western Electric Study (employees at the Hawthorne Works of the Western Electric Company in Chicago), those who initially completed the MMPI in 1957–58 were reexamined annually until 1967, primarily to determine the occurrence of new coronary heart disease events. The most recent follow–up for mortality was conducted in 1978. Researchers R.B. Shekelle, M. Gale, M.A. Ostfeld, and O. Paul used the Western Electric Study to investigate the relationship among hostility scores obtained at the initial examination, the subsequent 10–year incidence of coronary heart disease, and mortality after 20 years.[46] Overall, the odds of a major coronary heart disease event was 1.47 times greater for men with high hostility scores than for men with low hostility scores. That is, the 10–year incidence of major coronary events (myocardial infarction or coronary heart disease deaths) was greater for men with high hostility scores. Also, as illustrated in Figure 1–2, high levels of hostility were significantly and positively related to death from coronary heart disease after 20 years, as well as to death from malignant neoplasms and death from all causes combined. The MMPI hostility measure was also positively related to cigarette smoking, alcohol usage, and increasing age—the traditional risk factors for heart disease! In other words, individuals with high hostility scores were more likely to smoke cigarettes, drink alcoholic beverages, and be older in age.

Taken together, the findings from Duke Medical Center and those based on data from the Western Electric Study suggest that the tendency to endorse MMPI items reflective of hostility and possibly other dimensions of the AHA! Syndrome is an important risk factor for mortality from all causes and for CHD death. However, although the findings derived from these two studies were quite similar, another study reported by Edward McCranie and his colleagues at the Medical College of Georgia failed to show a significant relationship between the MMPI hostility scores and total mortality or coronary heart disease incidence.[48] These findings differed even though the characteristics of the sample (physicians who had completed the MMPI 25 years earlier at the time of the Medical College admission interview) and follow–up period were similar to those of the studies reported by John Barefoot and Richard Shekelle along with their respective associates. Furthermore, these two studies involving doctors were similar in that the samples of physicians were similar in age, attended state medical schools during the same era in the same geographic region, and experienced similar rates of CHD incidence and total mortality over the 25–year follow–up period.

Figure 1-2

Relation between MMPI hostility scores and risk of dying: 20–year follow–up

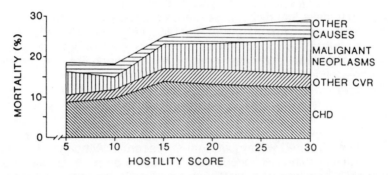

20–YEAR MORTALITY,

BY QUINTILE OF MMPI HOSTILITY SCORE,

WESTERN ELECTRIC STUDY, N=1877 MEN

Source: Reprinted with permission from Williams, R. B., Barefoot, J. C., and Shekelle, R. B. The health consequences of hostility, In Chesney, M.A. and Rosenman, R. H. (eds.), <u>Anger and Hostility i n Cardiovascular and Behavioral Disorders</u>, p. 178. New York: Hemisphere Publishing/McGraw–Hill, 1985.

Given the large similarities in these studies but the inconsistency in results, one is left wondering about whether the MMPI hostility measure is a consistent and reliable predictor of mortality across different population groups, or whether the relationship between hostility and mortality is too complex for the scale and might be shown to be more consistent if other dimensions of the AHA! Syndrome were evaluated. Then too, it is possible that the lack of a significant relationship between hostility and mortality in the McCranie study is due to other factors altogether. For example, the one crucial difference between the study by McCranie and the previous physician study is that the personality data (MMPI) in the McCanie study was collected from students applying for admission to medical school, rather than individuals already admitted. This difference could have significantly effected the results reported by McCranie and his colleagues. Furthermore, the pattern of scores obtained from scales that measured the test–taking attitudes of these individuals suggest that the applicants at the Medical College of Georgia were giving socially desirable answers to the questions, and not necessarily answers that really represented their state of emotional well–being.

Recently it has been acknowledged that the measure of hostility derived from the MMPI may not be a direct measure of Anger—Hostility–Aggression, but instead a measure of something else only related to the potential for hostility and anger. Current research focused on analysis of the items comprising the MMPI hostility measure has suggested that cynicism may be the fundamental construct it actually measures.[45,49] In fact, even a brief inspection of typical items in the scale—for example, Most people make friends because friends are likely to be useful to them; I have frequently worked under people who seem to have things arranged so that they get credit for good work but are able to pass off mistakes on to those under them—does make it sound like a measure of cynicism—defined as the belief that people are motivated in all their actions only by selfishness and a lack of basic trust in other people. Regardless of how we label it, however, high scores on this scale are predictive of adverse health consequences.

In fact, the extent to which cynicism and elements of the AHA! Syndrome are related will require further research. Although the nature of these relationships will undoubtedly turn out to be complex, the strong relationship between the MMPI measure and measures of anger, hostility, and Type–A behavior suggest that highly cynical individuals are likely to experience anger and hostility more often than individuals with a strong trust in other people. In an effort to clarify the meaning of the scale, Timothy Smith and Karl Frohm of the University of Utah conducted research and found that individuals with high cynicism-hostility scores are more prone to anger, more suspicious and resentful of others, experience more frequent and severe daily hassles, have fewer and less satisfactory supportive social interactions, and are likely to be manipulative in their social encounters.[49] To some extent, recent data that I have collected—although correlational in nature—also strongly support the notion that individuals with high scores on the MMPI hostility—cynicism measure experience feelings of anger more frequently and at a greater intensity across a wide range of social and interpersonal situations.[50] Given these observed relationships, it is tempting to speculate that adverse health consequences would also be notably worse for individuals with elevated scores on the various dimensions of anger (frequency, intensity, duration, suppression) as well as the MMPI hostility—cynicism measure. Although the studies that have been discussed do not lend themselves to more detailed analysis, I believe that we would profit tremendously if future research could determine whether different levels and combinations of the AHA! Syndrome are predictors of mortality from coronary heart disease and—especially—cancer.

The Tecumseh Community Health Study

The research that I have been a part of at the University of Michigan in Ann Arbor shows that certain dimensions of the AHA! Syndrome are indeed related to mortality from all causes combined.[51] Our study, directed from 1971 to 1983, by psychosocial epidemiologist Mara Julius, examined prospectively the relationship between anger–coping types, blood pressure, and mortality from all causes in a subsample of men and women age 30—69 from the Tecumseh Community Health Study, a longitudinal epidemiologic study of acute and chronic diseases throughout the whole community of Tecumseh, Michigan. The study started in 1957 and has collected data on several occasions since 1959. In fact, we have recently started to examine the health of the young adult offspring of individuals initially examined in 1959, and some of our findings will appear at other points in this book.[52,53]

In the study directed by Julius, adult respondents who said they were likely to suppress their anger in response to two potential anger–provoking situations had 1.7 times the mortality risk of those who expressed their anger. More specifically, respondents who suppressed their anger when unjustifiably confronted by their spouse had twice the mortality risk of those who expressed their anger. The mortality risk of those who suppressed anger when provoked by a person of authority (a policeman) was 1.2 times the mortality risk of those who expressed their anger. As is usual with any large–scale epidemiologic study, we found the relationships between suppressed anger and mortality to be invariant across age groups, gender, and educational levels, even when medical risk factors such as smoking, weight, blood pressure, and CHD status were considered. Moreover, as seen in Figure 1–3, suppressed anger significantly interacted with elevated blood pressure to predict the highest overall mortality risk. Persons who had elevated blood pressure and who scored high in suppressed anger were—on the average—five times more likely to have died during the 12–year follow–up compared with hypertensives who expressed their anger.

While several design limitations may have influenced the study results, the model of suppressed anger on which the measures were based is related to a specific conceptual model: Anger is induced by perceived unjust deprivation of a felt possession, such as one's rights. Unfortunately, there were only two situations (spouse disagreement, and provocation by a policeman) used to assess anger coping responses. This has been one of the study's greatest problems, along with using hypothetical situations as the focal point for determining complex Julius decided to examine the relationship between anger–coping types in the 192 marital pairs and mortality from all causes combined. The marital pairs were classified into groups by high and low scores in anger expression toward the spouse. The hypothetical situation involving disagreement with spouse was used—rather than the policeman—because we believe that, if the angry reactions associated with a provocation are consistent across many social situations and the attacks (verbal behavioral) are chronic—as from a spouse—then a state of resentment will arise. In this

Figure 1-3
Mortality rates in relation to suppressed anger responses and blood pressure scores: Tecumseh, Michigan, 1971–1983

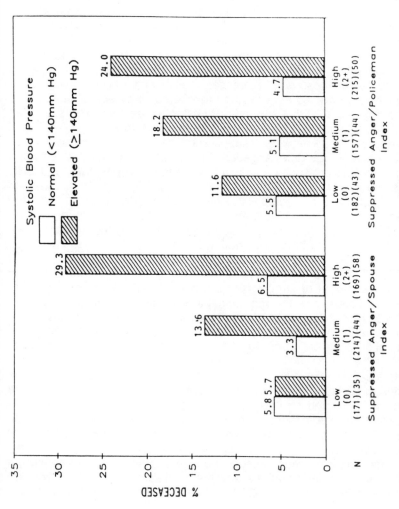

Source: Julius, M., Harburg, E., Cottington, E., and Johnson, E.H., Anger–coping types, blood pressure, and total mortality: A follow–up in Tecumseh, Michigan, 1971–1983. Reprinted with permission from *American Journal of Epidemiology*, 1988, p. 124:229.)

state, angry feelings and their physiological and biochemical processes are aroused by the hostile attitude that is maintained by the frequent and intense experience of anger. One would hope that the day–to–day interactions of most people are with an important significant other such as a spouse, rather than a policeman—but then, each of us marches to the beat of a different drummer. In any event, what Mara Julius discovered was that the lowest mortality rates were found when both husband and wife had low suppressed-anger scores. Moreover, the highest mortality rates were associated with there being a different pattern of anger–coping strategies between the husband and the wife. If both the husband and wife had high suppressed anger scores, these scores significantly predicted mortality for wives, but not for husbands.

Hostility, Mortality, and Ischemic Heart Disease in Finnish Men

It has been argued that one of the most convincing ways to support the notion that the AHA! Syndrome has adverse health consequences would be to replicate the pattern of results in various cultural groups. I am not sure if the rationale behind this notion has to do with the possibility that Americans are not good research volunteers (i.e., we give socially desirable responses to most psychological questionnaires) or that our health is so bad that any given factor at any given time will significantly predict poor health and mortality risk. Be this as it may, I have a very difficult time believing that we Americans will go out of our way for anything—let alone drop dead—so that there is proof for the notion that the AHA! Syndrome is deadly for your health. In any event, I want to turn your attention to the Finnish Study of Hostility and Ischemic Heart Disease.

The Finnish Study was prepared under the leadership of Markku Koskenvuo; it investigated the predictive association of hostility with ischemic heart disease during a 3-year follow–up in a population of 3,750 Finnish men, age 40—59 years.[55] Participants in the study were members of the Finnish Twin Cohort, a nationwide registry of adult twin pairs born in Finland before 1958. Although the questionnaires used to measure the AHA! Syndrome were somewhat different from those reported in other studies,[47,48,51,56] the findings are nevertheless quite interesting.

The 1981 twin study questionnaire included, in addition to medical history, several standard psychosocial questionnaire scales for assessing irritability, ease of anger–arousal, and argumentativeness. Using a combination of these variables to create a hostility measure, the sample of 3,750 Finnish men was divided into four groups according to level of hostility: (1) Most Hostile Group (188 men); (2) Hostile Group (376 men); (3) Medium or Moderate Hostile Group (1,938 men); and (4) Least Hostile Group (1,248 men). Even over the brief follow–up period of three years a greater number of men in the Most Hostile Group died compared with men in the other groups. The relative risk of mortality from all causes combined for the Most Hostile and Hostile Groups was 2.98, compared to 1.0 for the Least Hostile Group and 2.53 for the Medium Hostile Group. The relative risk of death from cardiovascular disease was 2.72 for the Most Hostile and Hostile Groups as compared to 1.0 for the Least Hostile Group and 2.09 for the Moderate Hostile Group. Moreover, the relative risk of mortality from violent means (i.e. homicides, suicides) was substantially greater for the Most Hostile and Hostile Groups (4.39) and Moderate Hostile Group (5.12), compared to 1.0 for the Least Hostile Group. Although the total number of deaths (65) was low after the three year follow–up period, a total of 109 men developed ischemic heart disease. Hostility did not predict ischemic heart disease among healthy men; but among the men with hypertension, the relative risk of ischemic heart disease was 12.9 for the Most Hostile Group, compared to 4.58 for the Moderate Hostile and Hostile groups and 1.0 for the Least Hostile Group. The team of investigators concluded that hostility is a strong determinant of mortality and coronary attack among hypertensive men with ischemic heart disease.

This study clearly demonstrated that the AHA! Syndrome is a useful and strong predictor of mortality and cardiovascular events. However, the mechanisms that explain the decreased survival among extremely hostile individuals can only be speculated. Much like research scientists in the United States, the group of Finnish investigators hypothesized that "stressful" stimuli may cause a "disbalance" in pituitary–adrenal and sympathetic–adrenal activity within hostile individuals. Whereas the pathophysiology underlying the development of ischemic heart disease and its manifestations such as sudden death, myocardial infarction, and angina pectoris are not totally understood, one of the basic mechanisms in most cases is coronary atherosclerosis. Myocardial infarction is usually preceded by coronary thrombosis of atherosclerotic plague, but the determinants that trigger these pathological events are poorly understood. Nevertheless, it is possible that extremely hostile individuals are more likely to engage in aggressive behaviors that somehow contribute to the development of fatal arrhythmias and coronary spasms. Interestingly enough, the findings of the Finnish study also showed a surprisingly strong association between the AHA! Syndrome and both heavy smoking and high cholesterol levels, both of which increase the risk of ischemic heart disease.

To summarize the relationship between the AHA! Syndrome and mortality, I would simply say that death is the bottom line. No matter how unimportant, exaggerated, or even false, these studies may be considered, the truth of the matter is that seeing red is better than being dead, but that seeing too much red contributes to early death from a variety of causes. Nevertheless, one of the major shortcomings of each of the studies reviewed in this section is a problem that social scientists refer to as the "direction of causality." In other words, it is conceivable that the causal relationship between the AHA! Syndrome and mortality may be somewhat different from the direction proposed.

Although it is the belief of most psychosomatic researchers—including myself—that the pendulum swings in the direction of the AHA! Syndrome being the initial event and the health problems and early mortality following, it is possible to have a relationship between two events without one causing changes in the other. For example, in the case of the relationship between obesity and health problems, it is possible that the onset of health problems leads to weight gain and obesity—rather than obesity being the cause of health problems. Another perspective on the relationship between obesity and health problems is that other factors referred to as "mediating events" are responsible for both weight gain and the onset of health problems. Is it possible that certain metabolic or endocrine factors constitute the sole cause of both conditions, or function as mediating factors in the relationship between obesity and physical illness? The relationship between the AHA! Syndrome and health problems can be similarly approached. I would even go so far as to say that it is probably true that certain mediating factors such as excessive smoking and alcohol usage, a poor diet rich in cholesterol, and excessive psychophysiological reactions to chronic stress do contribute to the relationship between the AHA! Syndrome and physical and emotional illness.

2

The Role of the AHA! Syndrome in Health and Psychological Well-being

After reading through Chapter 1, you should have no great difficulty with the notion that the AHA! Syndrome is deadly. But then again, what exactly does being intensely angry for a prolonged period of time over a situation where it is best to suppress rather than express these feelings, say, have to do with *your* health? The answer to this question is much, and I will do my best in later chapters to present you with the research evidence that convinced me the AHA! Syndrome is bad for both physical and mental health. Before getting into the very complex and involved undertaking of linking the AHA! Syndrome to specific health problems, however, I wish to explain somewhat generally the possible ways it leads to poor health.

Apart from purely biological and physiological responses related to the experience of anger and hostility, the mechanisms that relate the AHA! Syndrome and health problems are thought to involve negative health behaviors and practices—smoking, alcohol intake, lack of exercise, and so forth. For example, in the Finnish Study of Hostility and Ischemic Heart Disease, hostile individuals tended to be heavy smokers and to have higher cholesterol levels. Similarly, high levels of hostility were positively associated with cigarette smoking and alcohol use among respondents in the Western Electric Study. Therefore, one explanation that provides some insight into the relationship between the AHA! Syndrome and health problems is that angry and hostile individuals are more likely to smoke cigarettes, drink alcohol, and possibly engage in other behaviors (e.g., maintain poor dietary, sleep, and exercise habits) that increase the risk of health problems and subsequent mortality. The basic problem with this explanation is that the association between the AHA! Syndrome and mortality were reported to be unchanged when known risk factors or potential mediating factors such as cigarette smoking, alcohol consumption, weight, and even cholesterol levels among the men in the Finnish Twin Study were taken into consideration. Although it is quite possible that known risk factors may contribute to the worsening of health problems among highly angry and hostile individuals, the association between mortality and the AHA! Syndrome is apparently independent of the standard risk factors.

Another explanation that is more physiological in nature is based on the pattern of physiological responses generated by what is referred to as the "defense reaction" or the "fight/flight" response. This pattern, as described by physician and researcher Redford Williams, is characterized by increased pumping of blood by the heart, shunting of this increased cardiac output away from the skin and abdominal viscera to the skeletal musculature and increased secretion of norepinephrine, epinephrine, cortisol, and prolactin.[1] Moreover, the defense reaction is provoked in situations where the individual perceives either a sense of threat and danger or a strong need for continuous mental effort to understand and cope with the stressful situations.

Could it be that the physiological concomitants of this defense reaction are so similar to the bodily reactions during the experience of anger that the two are inseparable? My answer to this question is yes. Remember that anger—much like the defense reaction—is elicited and provoked by social situations wherein the individual perceives (1) a loss or threat of loss of (2) something felt to be possessed, through (3) perceived arbitrary acts by others. The experience of chronic anger is thought to increase the heart rate and the blood pressure and to provide blood for the muscles needed to engage in an attack or to defend against the loss of one's highly valued possessions. There is also a strong outpouring of hormones (noradrenaline, cortisol, and testosterone) into the body. Individuals who have a strong disposition to experience frequent and intense feelings of anger and who are ineffective in managing and/or expressing their anger probably engage in more behaviors reminiscent of the defense reaction. Such individuals would be expected to experience more anger in daily life as a result of hostile attitudes. Therefore, angry and hostile individuals are also believed to experience greater secretions of norepinephrine, epinephrine, and cortisol during the experience of anger,which—as indicated above—is expected to occur with greater frequency and intensity among highly hostile individuals.

Much like the fight/flight reaction, the experience of intense anger elevates blood pressure and heart rate as well as increases muscle tension and respiration rate. How are the fight/flight reaction and the physiological reactions associated with the AHA! Syndrome related to illness? In the case of the neuroendocrine reactivity involved in anger, there occurs a sequence of events that is thought to be of importance in atherogenesis since cortisol is known to potentiate both the cardiovascular and metabolic effects of catecholamines (norepinephrine and epinephrine), which could accelerate processes involved in "endothelial injury"—the most widely accepted model of atherogenesis. Support for the notion that cortisol worsens or possibly accelerates the atherogenic process can be gleaned from studies reported by K. Kalbak and by R.G. Troxler and associates.[2,3] In the study by Kalbak, the administration of corticosteroids was directly related to acceleration of atherosclerosis in patients with rheumatoid arthritis, while Troxler and associates showed that patients with more severe angiographically documented coronary artery disease have higher cortisol levels during the early morning (9:00 a.m.) than patients with lower levels of coronary artery disease. Several recent studies have also reported findings supportive of a pathogenic role of testosterone in atherosclerosis. For example, a study published by E.L. Klaiber and associates showed that male heart attack victims have higher levels of plasma estradiol (an estrogenic hormone), compared to men who have no evidence of coronary disease.[4] This observation gains some added importance when one considers the fact that most of the plasma estradiol in men is derived from testosterone by a conversion process referred to as "aromatization," which is stimulated or partially set in motion by norepinephrine.[5,6]

In view of the growing body of research showing that "stress" is related to a depression or dysregulation of immune system functioning, a similar chain of events may contribute to carcinogenesis by disrupting the immune function necessary for reducing or rejecting tumors among individuals with high levels of anger and hostility. But then again, it is also possible that the dysfunction necessary for tumor formation may be set in motion by the overindulgence in negative health practices (e.g., smoking cigarettes, alcohol consumption, high cholesterol diets) or high levels of anger and hostility. Furthermore, the increased cancer mortality connected to hostility in the Western Electric Study, for example, could be related to the findings of Drs. P. Graves and C.B. Thomas in the Johns Hopkins cancer precursors study, which showed that future cancer victims have disturbed and unsatisfactory early relationships with their parents as well as a relative lack of well-balanced pattern in their personal interactions.[7] These characteristics could contribute to individual differences in the experience and expression of anger and hostility as well as other dimensions of the AHA! Syndrome. However, no matter how much we psychologists convince ourselves of the importance of supportive links with family and the susceptibility to illness, and no matter how strong the evidence connecting the AHA! Syndrome and disturbed relationships and illness, the ultimate linkage between the AHA! Syndrome and illness must involve dysregulations in one or several physiological systems.

As it stands, the operation of most physiological systems is maintained by what is referred to as "homeostasis" which was first described as a principle by the French physiologist Claude Bernard (1813–78) who is generally considered to be the father of experimental medicine. Homeostasis is the obtainment of a relatively stable state of equilibrium or balance in the physiological and hormonal systems that control our bodily functions. Any condition that disrupts the balance or the steady state will automatically set in motion countermeasures to restore the balance. More than a trillion cells race through the blood stream and lymph system—for example—searching for invaders or antigens, be they bacteria, viruses, fungi, or the body's own cells gone awry (as in tumor or cancer cells). Furthermore, these lymphocytes identify each antigen and produce antibodies that reach out and destroy it. In this sequence of events, phagocytes finish the fight and literally clean the battlefield of all debris. They are aided by another clean-up crew referred to as macrophages, which are important for healing wounds and infections. These "macrophages," which actually ingest invading foreign bodies, have been shown to be affected by our level of stress and emotional state.

The immune system is set in motion in the first place by natural killer (NK) cells which act as an early-warning surveillance system against cancer cells and the spread of tumors. In addition to natural killer cells, lymphocytes, phagocytes, and macrophages, there are also cells in the immune system called "T helper cells" and "T suppression cells," which help regulate and maintain the balance and homeostasis of the immune response. The T helper (or inducer) cells encourage another group of cells—called "B cells"—to generate antibody-producing plasma cells. Remember that antibodies attack the invading bodies—antigens. On the other hand, T suppressor (or cytotoxic) cells inhibit the formation of antibodies. Thus, there is a balance or steady state in the immune response maintained in part by the ratio of T helper and T suppressor cells.

When the immune system gets out of balance and overreacts to exogenous agents, it is highly probable that the body will react by developing an allergy. If, however, the immune system underreacts to outside or exogenous agents, the reaction of the body is likely to be the development of a severe chronic infection. In any case, the system is constantly fluctuating in its quest for the steady state. For example, a prospective study of occupational stress among healthy tax accountants that was conducted by B. Dorian and colleagues revealed that the differences in certain immune parameters between the accountants and a control group changed with time (NK activity being highest when the ratio of helper to suppressor T cells was lower).[8] Interestingly enough, the accountants and the controls experienced no difference in the number of stressful events, but the accountants suffered more distress—depression, irritability, anxiety, and somatic symptoms.

In other recent studies, the stress of attending medical school on students immune measures has been examined.[9-11] The general organization of these studies is that immune measures obtained before the academic exams are compared to measures obtained over the course of the year as the students undergo academic stress. In this context, several studies have revealed a reduction in NK cell activity and declines in the number of helper T cells in their ratio to suppressor T cells— reductions that were lowest in students with the greatest levels of stress.

A recent study directed by Ronald Glaser investigated the clinical significance of such changes over the course of a year.[10] The results revealed that there were significant decrements in production by mitogen-stimulated lymphocytes of gamma interferon—an antiviral factor—along with higher titers of antibody to Epstein-Barr virus, suggesting activation of a latent virus and therefore weaker cell-mediated immunity. More importantly, the incidence of self-reported symptoms of infectious illness rose during examinations which led the investigators to propose a connection between stress, suppression of cellular immunity, and viral infection.

Another example that is often used to explain the homeostatic mechanism involves the control of body temperature. Most biochemical and physiological reactors function most efficiently at 98.6 degrees Fahrenheit within the body, although there are some reactions that operate better at lower or higher temperatures. Sperm, for example, require a temperature below 98.6 degrees; they are destroyed at body temperature. This is why the sperm are produced and stored in testicles that hang in a scrotal sac outside the body. And the scrotum has an automatic reaction to temperature changes. For example, in hot weather or when bodily heat has increased due to exercise, physical exertion, or a hot shower, the scrotum expands and the testes are automatically lowered away from the body. By contrast, the scrotal sac contracts when a man enters a cold environment such as a cold shower. The testes are brought closer to the body for warmth and protection. In a similar manner, body temperature and the metabolic rate are increased automatically to help overcome invasions by infectious organisms. In this case, the resultant fever is part of the homeostatic maneuver necessary for fighting the disease.

Extending the notion of homeostasis I believe that the emotions comprising the AHA! Syndrome may also operate in a similar manner. In other words, the adrenaline-mediated fight/flight response initially described by Walter B. Cannon in 1929—involving blood pressure and heart rate increases, skeletal muscle vasodilation, visceral vasoconstriction, and biological changes associated with energy mobilization—may be inappropriately managed in our modern-day world.[12] These physiologic and metabolic changes are merely reflections of the brain's automatic control of the body's functions, and are appropriate for maintaining the homeostatic balance of the human organism. However, what is inappropriate in our "civilized" society is the tremendous psychological and self-imposed effort demanded in order to survive and be successful. In other words, our brains are appropriately making adjustments to maintain homeostasis, but the environment in which we live is in a severe state of dysregulation. Therefore, we should not be surprised at the extent of anger and hostility in these times. I am not saying that it is right or that it is wrong to be angry. The big problem is that it may not be possible to restore balance in the modern world. If so, the anger that we experience and express is a completely useless and wearily repetitious exercise in futility.

Could it be that no matter how angry we feel—about being stuck in rush-hour traffic, or the realization that our oceans have become so polluted that medical supplies are washing up on the shores of some of our major cities—there will be no immediate or automatic or long-term response on our part that is capable of restoring balance? But, then again, we did land a man (and more that one) on the moon, and we did successfully piece together the Challenger space shuttle and the story of its disastrous end. Maybe—just maybe—we can find a way to regulate this unbalanced world of ours, which automatically elicits biological and psychological homeostatic mechanisms that erode our well-being and health and destroys our sense of dignity and pride.

In any case, it is highly plausible that the AHA! Syndrome contributes to poor health, and the mechanisms involved deserve much more research attention.

THE ASSOCIATION BETWEEN ANGER AND PSYCHOLOGICAL DISTRESS

Among the great majority of psychoanalytic theorists, anger and hostility are thought to be important contributors to the development of depression. For example, in 1911 Karl Abraham hypothesized that anger and hostility associated with the death and loss of a spouse or a significant loved one become self-directed through identification with the beloved, and contribute to the onset of depression.[13] A few years later, Sigmund Freud added that strong feelings of remorse, guilt, and shame over a loss trigger a need to suffer, as well as a lowering of self-esteem and one's ability to function. Ultimately, this was believed to cause a self-directed or inward hostility and depressed mood (see Chapter 1).

Although there is strong evidence for an association between anger-hostility and depression, the position taken by many modern-day psychologists is that the occurrence of one of these emotions does not necessarily mean that the other must be experienced by the individual. Nevertheless, feelings of hopelessness and depression may be the end result or one sequel to the unsuccessful use of anger as an impetus to change something that is wrong. This is the case of many young black Americans, who eventually begin to feel helpless and depressed about their lack of control over important resources that are necessary to achieve upward social, educational, and economic mobility. There is an eventual giving up or "learned helplessness", as psychologist Martin Seligman has labelled this process of dealing with uncontrollable bad events.[14] Learned helplessness causes a collapse of effort, and the development of a pessimistic style and perception that there are no actions or solutions to the problem. There also occurs a realization that the frequent experience of intense anger about the problem will have no impact on its demise. In the case of individuals who are seriously depressed, they have given up hope and abandoned all the usual mechanisms of coping. They perceive themselves as neither capable of initiating actions necessary for adaptation, nor worthy of surviving the crisis situation.

As indicated earlier, I believe that anger and other elements of the AHA! Syndrome are part of the basic fight/flight response pattern that is elicited during times of stress. Their occurrence can be viewed as being the first line of defense in reaction to threat, ensuring our survival. If so, then the simple notion that depression is turned inward makes more than a little sense. It lends support to the argument that anger is a natural response acting as a signal when something is wrong or out of balance. In the case of depression, the angry and hostile state is a complex psychobiophysiologic reaction informing the person that something about the self is wrong, out of balance, and in a state of dysregulation.

Research by psychologist Martin Seligman and his associates at the University of Pennsylvania has been quite influential and instrumental in uncovering the ways of responding to uncontrollable bad events that contribute to learned helplessness and depression.[15,16] According to Seligman's reformulation of the learned helplessness model, individuals with a explanatory style—the habitual way in which people explain negative and bad events—that is pessimistic are more likely to display helplessness when confronted with a negative event than individuals with an optimistic explanatory style. In other words, persons who habitually construe the causes of negative or bad events as internal ("it's my fault"), stable ("it's going to last forever"), and global ("it's going to ruin and undermine everything I do") are probably—when they experience negative and stressful life events—more susceptible to feeling helpless and depressed than persons with the opposite style. For the most part, a review of the research literature uncovers strong evidence of the predicted relationship between the pessimistic explanatory style and increased depression. Furthermore, a recent study by Christopher Peterson, Martin Seligman, and George Vaillant showed that explanatory style—as extracted from responses to questionnaires completed by 99 graduates of the Harvard University class in 1942–44—predicted poor health 35 years later.[16] In fact, the pessimistic explanatory style predicted poor health at ages 45 through 60 even when physical and mental health at age 25 were controlled. Although the mechanisms by which pessimistic explanatory style increases the risk of poor health (e.g., accumulated negative life events; loneliness and depression; increased immunosuppression; alcohol abuse or smoking) are not known, the findings of this study show that pessimism in early adulthood appears to be a risk factor for poor health in middle and late adulthood.

Depression is an extreme form of psychological distress and bears little or no relationship to the layman's concept of "feeling depressed," "feeling down", or "feeling blue." Clinical depression is actually considered to be one of the most profound psychiatric illness; the individual experiencing it tends to be quite pessimistic about the future in general and more specifically about the likelihood of overcoming future problems. Feelings of guilt, irritability, anxiety, restlessness, self-deprecation, loss of appetite, and sleeping disturbances are common. Other symptoms include crying, refusal to speak, psychomotor retardation, physical complaints, and weakness, fatigue, or loss of energy. Depression is a very complicated set of reactions; it reduces the affect of the individual, constricts behavior and thought, and severely limits the individual's capability to cope and function in a wide variety of situations. To a great extent, depressed individuals suffer from a delusional and diminished view of their intellectual capacity to function rationally in the world around them. In these instances, the depression is unbearable to the degree that such individuals become very overcontrolled and tend to deny their own impulses, thoughts, and reactions to events. The person then does his or her most to avoid unpleasantness and will make major concessions in order to avoid confrontations.

On the biological side, depression is thought to be the result of specific biochemical dysfunctions. As it turns out, some of the most important biochemical and hormonal markers of depression—norepinephrine for instance—are the same ones believed to be related to the fight/flight response and the exaggerated experience of anger and hostility. Thus, apparently there is nothing wrong with the view that depression represents intense anger turned inward against the self. There may be a problem, however, on the insistence of psychoanalysis in forming a causal relationship where depression is viewed as being caused solely by anger turned inward. In my view, depression is a multifaceted and highly complicated set of mechanisms that effect severe limitations in behavioral, cognitive, and emotional functioning to the point that the individual sees himself or herself as neither capable of initiating actions necessary for survival nor worthy of surviving. Anger is the label we have assigned to one of the basic emotions elicited during times of threat. Anger is a basic component in the early-warning system that ensures our survival and protects us from events and circumstances physically and emotionally harmful to our survival. In the case of depression, anger may be the initial response in an unspecified sequence of events whose aim is to restore balance to the self when it is in a state of dysregulation.

If depression were caused simply by anger that is repressed and turned inward, we would expect clinically depressed patients not to express their anger and hostility outwardly. As it turns out, this is a myth. Most depressed patients spend a good part of a therapy hour expressing feelings of anger, irritability and hostility. In one study of a group of depressed women that was reported by Paul Wender and Donald Klein, anger and hostility not only increased during episodes of acute depression, but also continued after these episodes.[17] Thus on the one hand, it is by all means possible that serious depression represents an attempt to turn feelings of anger and other strong emotions inward. On the other hand, depressed patients not only express feelings of anger and hostility; they also tend to experience an increase in the intensity and severity of anger and hostility. To a certain extent, findings of this type indicate that talking about anger or talking out anger is an effective manner for an individual to get in touch with feelings that are repressed and possibly related to depression.

Although we are only beginning to determine how clinically depressed patients respond to our new self-report measures of the experience and expression of anger, studies of the relationship between depression and anger in college student samples provide confirmation of the complex interrelationships between the experience and expression of emotions. For example, it is common to find a positive relationship between high levels of depression, anger, and anxiety. In other words, persons who experience high levels of depression also experience high levels of anger and anxiety. Also, one of my recent studies strongly indicated that intense depression, anxiety, and anger can characterize both individuals who habitually suppress anger as well as those who habitually express anger outwardly.[18] Interesting in this regard are findings from other studies that high levels of both suppressed and expressed anger are related to physical disorders and to mortality from all causes combined.

So there you have it, and the complete truth is that it is not terribly important whether anger and depression are related. I think there is good evidence for their coexistence, but the degree to which the experience, expression, or control of anger is present in depression and other forms of psychological distress could be discussed from now until the cows come home. One's interpretation of the relationship between anger (suppressed anger in particular) and depression will depend on the circumstances and events that trigger these emotions in a particular individual, as well as that individual's appraisal of those circumstances and the experience of other emotions.

Before moving away from discussion of the relationship between anger and depression, let me share certain observations and findings regarding the relationship between anger and health problems that we obtained from the National Survey of Black Americans (NSBA) conducted in 1979–80. The NSBA was directed by social psychologist James Jackson at the University of Michigan; and it represented the first nationally representative, cross-sectional mental health survey of the adult (18 years and older) black population.[19] Its sample of 2,107 adults was assembled in such a way as to ensure that every black household would have an equal probability of selection. In the NSBA, the measure of anger expression was obtained only for those respondents who reported experiencing a "personal problem" that caused them to feel they were at "the point of a nervous breakdown." Subjects responded to a series of items asking them to report how they coped with the personal problem. The anger items (e.g., Did you lose your temper? Did you fight or argue with other people?) pertinent to this discussion assessed the frequency with which anger was expressed outwardly at people and objects in the environment during the period that the respondent experienced the personal problem. In addition to examining the NSBA anger coping measure, the present discussion will focus on a number of physician-diagnosed health problems (arthritis, ulcers, cancer, hypertension, diabetes, liver difficulties, kidney problems, stroke, circulatory problems in the arms or legs, and sickle-cell disease) relatively common to black Americans.

Reviewing the NSBA data, Clifford Broman and I discovered that respondents who experienced a high level of outwardly expressed anger had a substantially higher number of health problems than their peers who expressed low and moderate levels of anger or those who experienced other emotional reactions.[20,21] Also—much like the study of hostility and ischemic heart disease and mortality in Finnish twins (see Chapter 1)—anger expression among black Americans was significantly related to cigarette smoking and heavy consumption of alcohol. Whereas anger expressed outwardly was related to these negative health behaviors—which increase the risk of health problems—the relationship between anger expression and the actual number of health problems was found to be independent of smoking and drinking problems as well as age, gender, and whether the respondents lived in a large urban city or small towns in rural America. The only factor that changed the relationship between health problems and high levels of outwardly expressed anger had to do with employment status. Respondents who were unemployed (and 43 percent of the NSBA respondents were unemployed at the time of the study) were more likely to have a higher number of health problems if anger was expressed outwardly at a high level.

Broman and I concluded overall that black Americans at increased risk for health problems may be identified by how often they experience and express anger during periods of emotional distress, and also that an excessive amount of life strain makes the situation worse. In this regard, our findings from the NSBA data were remarkably similar to those for both blacks and whites in the Detroit Study of hypertension and suppressed hostility that was directed by Ernest Harburg.[22,23] In this study of more than 1,000 adult men and women the relationship between suppressed hostility and hypertension was mediated by the degree of "job strain" and "family strain" as well as by "socio-ecological environmental stress."[24,25] Blood pressure was highest in persons with high levels of job strain and who had a tendency to suppress angry feelings when provoked as shown in Figure 2-1.

Persons who experienced high levels of family stress did not have high blood pressure if they openly expressed their anger; this effect is seen in Figure 2-2.

STRESS AND THE AHA! SYNDROME

Figure 2-1
Anger-coping style, job strain, and blood pressure: The Detroit Study

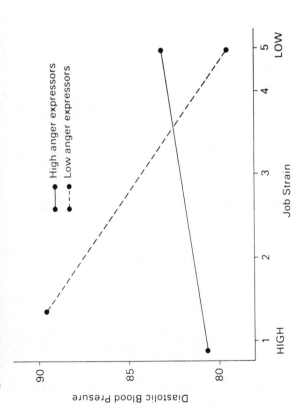

Source: Reprinted with permission from Gentry, W.D. Relationship of anger-coping styles and blood pressure among black Americans. In Chesney, M.A. and Rosenman, R.H. (eds.), Anger and Hostility in Cardiovascular and Behavioral Disorders, p. 144. Washington, D.C.: Hemisphere Publishing/McGraw-Hill, 1985.

Figure 2-2
Anger-coping style, family strain, and blood pressure: The Detroit Study

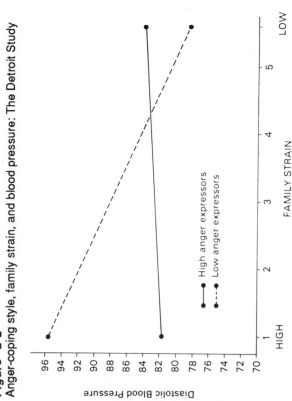

Source: Reprinted with permission from Gentry, W.D. Relationship of anger-coping styles and blood pressure among black Americans. In Chesney, M.A. and Rosenman R.H. (eds)., Anger and Hostility in Cardiovascualr and Behavioral Disorders, p. 144. Washington, D.C.: Hemisphere Publishing/McGraw-Hill, 1985.

The concept of "stress" is a very difficult scientific construct. There has been a wealth of research directed at understanding the nature and impact of stress on illness. As Hans Selye—a pioneer in stress research—pointed out some years ago, "stress is a scientific concept which has suffered from the mixed blessing of being too well known and too little understood."[26] Although there have been numerous models and definitions, the model most frequently cited as the first serious attempt to link stress to illness is that proposed by Selye in 1956. As a medical student, he had observed that many diseases present themselves with a number of common characteristics. Regardless of the physical disorder, patients would often complain of diffuse pains in their joints and muscles, intestinal disturbances with loss of appetite, loss of weight, and a general sense of physical discomfort.

Later working as a physician and scientist, Selye was able to reproduce these clinical manifestations of stress in laboratory rats by injecting a variety of toxic substances. The results of these studies led Selye to the notion that a certain amount of nonspecific damage to the organism is superimposed on the specific characteristics of any and all diseases. Based on these observations and the fact that certain nonspecific curative measures, provided by physicians (such as encouraging patients to get more rest and take it easy) are useful and therapeutic in treating patients with a wide variety of diseases, Selye hypothesized the existence of a general nonspecific reaction pattern on the part of the organism in response to threat or damage. Seyle also thought that this nonspecific response is absolutely necessary to the body's mobilization against threats to homeostasis. Following a series of studies—primarily involving animals—Selye proposed a general theory of stress through which he attempted to describe a nonspecific response pattern involving emotional and neurohormonal changes.

In the   model proposed by Selye, "stress" is defined as a nonspecific response of the body to any demand made on it, be that demand negative (e.g., death of spouse,loss of job) or positive (e.g., getting married,being promoted). Selye referred to this nonspecific pattern of exposure to stressors as the general adaptation syndrome (GAS). The GAS was conceptualized as evolving through three stages: (1) alarm reaction (2) resistance and (3) exhaustion. The alarm reaction is the most rapid component observed in response to a specific threat to homeostasis. During the "alarm reaction", there is a strong release of epinephrine along with a high level of physiological arousal (e.g., elevated blood pressure, surges in heart rate and hormones) and of negative emotions such as anxiety and depression, mood changes, and feelings of discomfort and doom. Does this sound familiar? Could this be the fight or flight response? In any case, during the alarm reaction, there is a tremendous vulnerability to increases in intensity of the specific threats and to other extraneous stressors. In the extreme, there is a heightened susceptibility to infections and illness; and if the nature of the stress and its accompanying negative emotional responses are severe enough and unavoidable, death occurs within a short time (hours or days) after initiation of the alarm reaction. However, if the stress or nature of threat is less severe and if there is prolonged exposure, certain mechanisms within GAS (probably through pituitary adrenocorticotropic hormones or ACTH) stimulates initiation of the resistance stage.

During "resistance", physiological arousal and hormonal activity remain at a high level, but decrease somewhat through adaptation. In essence, the parasympathetic branch of the autonomic nervous system attempts to counteract or balance the strong discharges from the sympathetic nervous system and thus restore the irregularities to homeostasis. During resistance, the organism is capable of enduring and coping with the particular stressor(s) and to resist further debilitating effects. On the other hand, the threshold for eliciting the alarm reaction is substantially lowered, so that there is a heightened sensitivity to new stressors and events that would threaten homeostasis. In the case of extreme exposure to the stressor(s) at intense levels and/or for a prolonged period of time, there is a depletion of the hormonal reserves; fatigue sets in; and eventually the organism enters the final stage of GAS, which is referred to as "exhaustion". During this stage, there is a decreased ability of the organism to resist either the original stressor or extraneous stressors, and the negative affect experienced during this phase is much like the clinical depression discussed in the previous section.

As to the AHA! Syndrome considered from the perspective of Selye's general adaptation syndrome, it is quite possible that the state of resistance might be maintained and prolonged either as long as hostility is repressed and remains subconscious, or else as long as the conscious experience of hostility is exacerbated by frequent and intense anger from new or repeated stimuli. If this latter situation of continual stress does occur, however, it could precipitate an adaptation crisis that might lead to the last stage of the GAS: the state of exhaustion. As indicated above, resistance can no longer be sustained during the state of exhaustion, and there follows a cessation of active emotional reactions that is brought about by a withdrawal from reality, chronic pessimism and depression, and regression to paranoid attitudes as a way of coping with the situation. In the case of anger, the state of resistance and adaptation will never break down following a short alarm reaction. Although there may be problems with adaptation to the circumstances, the single anger episode is generally short-lived, and the individual never gets to the stage of exhaustion. However, if anger is transmuted into chronic hostility and aggression or inadequately repressed from consciousness, the individual will have tremendous difficulty in regaining physiological and emotional homeostasis.

Although there are various models and theories of stress, each theory eventually leans heavily on two components that are not necessarily so very unrelated to each other. The first is the involvement of the fight/flight response in the initial phase of the reaction to threats to survival. The second is that—regardless of the importance that the theory places on stress or psychological factors as precursors of illness—the final pathway between stress and disease is likely to involve physiologic and biochemical factors associated with hyperarousal of autonomic nervous system functioning when it occurs in excess.

Be that as it may, there is enough evidence to indicate that anger and other elements of the AHA! Syndrome contribute either directly or indirectly to frequent and heightened activations of the sympathetic nervous system. The excessive activation is thought to be associated with both acute (in this case, infectious) and chronic diseases. Whereas it is extremely difficult to design the type of study that would delineate each of the components in the stress—AHA! Syndrome—illness continuum, a number of investigative studies are nevertheless relevant to the present discussion.

The first study to be discussed here is the work by Daniel H. Funkenstein, Stanley H. King, and Margaret E. Drolette that was summarized in a book called Mastery of Stress, published in 1957.[27]

Their study involved a series of experiments with a group of college men, carried out over a two-year period at Harvard University. The study focused on emotional and physiological reactions to stress during laboratory experiments administered at weekly intervals. Particular emphasis was placed on two phases of the stress reaction: (1) the acute, immediate reaction; and (2) the ability to master, or failure to master, stress on a time continuum. From an emotional point of view, the acute reactions of the 125 young men were of three main types, each of which had its characteristic physiological reaction: (1) anger directed outward, associated with a norepinephrine-like pattern; (2) anger directed inward— associated with a epinephrine-like pattern; and (3) anxiety—accompanied by epinephrine-like patterns.

In the laboratory stress experiments, the men were deliberately frustrated in their efforts to solve difficult computational problems. For example, imagine yourself the subject in an experiment and being told that most people can solve the problems in ten minutes—when in reality there is not sufficient time. Imagine also that while you are attempting to solve the problem you are being criticized and hassled by the examiner just enough to make you feel irritated and angry, but not enough that it is obvious the examiner is trying to pull your strings and get you mad as hell. In other words, the situation is so ambiguous that you could either blame the examiner for your failures or else place the blame on yourself. This is how the Harvard experiment was set up: Its effect was to hinder the subject and threaten his feelings of self-worth and self-regard, without actually preventing him from solving the problems.

One of the most unique aspects of this study was the interview with the subjects that took place at the end of the stress-testing session. From the responses and reactions given, it was possible to categorize the types of feelings reported. Responses were coded to determine the extent that the subject's emotions about the situation were directed toward the experimenter and the general situation, or directed inwardly toward himself and his inability to solve the problems. Although many of today's psychosomatic scientists recognize only that two predominant anger-coping patterns—anger directed outwardly at the examiner, and directing anger inwardly toward oneself—emerged from this research, several other response patterns were exhibited by the subjects.

Basically, there were seven psychological-emotional coping styles elicited by the exposure to stressful events in the Harvard study, plus a final category reserved for men who did not fit neatly into the other categories.

1.   Predominantly Anger-Out: largely characterized by the experience of anger as well as some anxiety, in which the direction of anger was either outward or mostly outward (34 students)

2.   Predominantly Anger-In: all men classified as only experiencing anger or some anxiety as well, in which the direction of the anger was either inward or mostly inward but partly outward (31 students)

3.   Anger Equal in Direction: largely characterized by the experience of anger and some anxiety in which the direction of anger was equally outward and inward (3 students)

4.   Performance Anxiety: all cases in which the major emotion reported was performance anxiety, regardless of the experience of any minor emotion (2 students)

5.   Severe anxiety: all men classified as experiencing severe anxiety, regardless of any minor emotion (23 students)

6.   Equal Anger and Anxiety: characterized by the experience of both anger and anxiety, with neither emotional reaction being dominant (12 students).

7.   No Emotion Reported: no emotion experienced during the stress-testing session (15 students)

8.   Miscellaneous: all men not classifiable under any of the above conditions (5 students)

As can be observed, a variety of emotional reactions were reported in response to the laboratory stressors. Certainly, the most frequent and predominant response was anger, with an almost equal number of subjects being classified as Anger-In and Anger-Out. However, the experience of emotional responses is a continuous process wherein a variety of reactions and behaviors occur. Classification of the responses into these seven categories only represents an attempt to capture the dominant personality style. As it turns out, Funkenstein and his colleagues anticipated the difficulties associated with identifying an individual's habitual emotional reactions to stress from limited observations made in the laboratory. To validate their "diagnosis," they obtained a second measure of each subject's emotional reactivity by interviewing the subject's roommate. Neither the roommate nor the interviewer had any knowledge of how the subject reacted in the laboratory. Interestingly enough, there was large agreement between the roommates' evaluations of the subjects' emotional reactions during real-life stresses and the classification of the subjects' emotional reactions to stress in the laboratory.

So, the predominant emotional responses were: (1) anger directed outward (27 percent of the subjects); (2) anger directed inward (25 percent of the subjects); or (3) anxiety (20 percent of the subjects). Together, 72 percent of the subjects (90 out of the 125 men) were classified as having one of these three dominant emotional response styles when confronted with laboratory and real-life stress. The study clearly demonstrated the usefulness of investigating emotional reactions to stress in the laboratory. But what knowledge was gained about the ability of the young men to handle stress? What about the relationship between the emotional reactivity to stress and those physiological reactions thought to represent the basic disposition that is predictive of psychosomatic illness. What did Funkenstein and his colleagues really learn about the fight/flight reaction and the ability of individuals to handle stress over time?

From a physiological standpoint, men who were classified as having a predominantly Anger-Out coping style to stress experienced a low intensity of physiological activity during the stress and had an excessive secretion of a norepinephrine-like substance. Anger-In and Severe Anxiety were both accompanied by a high intensity of physiological reactivity during the stress, and these subjects exhibited an excessive secretion of an epinephrine-like substance. Furthermore, the Severe Anxiety Group had a more intense physiological reaction than the Anger-In Group, while the physiology of the No Emotion Group was remarkably similar too that of the Anger-Out Group—low intensity of physiological reactions, and excessive secretion of a norepinephrine-like substance.

The finding that the Anger-Out and No Emotion Groups were similar in their physiological reactions to stress suggests that these two emotional reaction styles represent more efficient ways of coping with stress than Severe Anxiety and Anger-In. As it turns out, the men who reported Severe Anxiety performed poorly on the tasks, while those who reported Anger-In had good performance and those who reported Anger-Out or No Emotion had excellent performance. The explanation for this finding may rest in the fact that norepinephrine, which is the sympathetic neurotransmitter emanating mainly from sympathetic nerve endings in vascular walls throughout the body, evokes almost no generalized physiological response other than increasing peripheral resistance. On the other hand, epinephrine—or, as it is also known, adrenaline—which is derived almost exclusively from adreno-medullary secretion, is released during events that necessitate an emergency reaction. Therefore, the men who reacted with either Anger-In or Severe Anxiety evoked an emergency physiological reaction, whereas those men not bothered emotionally and those who were upset emotionally and reacted with Anger-Out did not evoke an emergency fight/flight response to the stress.

One of the reasons behind this pattern of physiological reactivity is the psychological difference between Anger-Out and either Anger-In or Severe Anxiety: In Anger-Out, the emotional and psychological discharge is expressed outward—away from the self and ego. In essence, the threat to psychological homeostasis is blamed on others rather than the self. In contrast, both Anger-In and Severe Anxiety blame the threat to homeostasis on the self, which is also the object of the threat. In the case of the Severe Anxiety reaction, anxiety may also represent the subject's fear of possible retaliation by others (the examiners, in this case) for his hostile and aggressive thoughts against them.

Although the Anger-Out, Anger-In, and Severe Anxiety Groups differed in their performance of difficult laboratory tasks, no relationship was found between the type of acute reaction exhibited by subjects and their subsequent handling of the stressful situation as monitored physiologically. In fact, just as many men whose initial reaction was Anger-Out, Anger-In, or Severe Anxiety eventually either mastered the stress or failed to master it. In other words, the Anger-Out, Anger-In, and Severe Anxiety respondents all had an equally good chance of adapting to and mastering the stress.

Extended analysis reveals, then, that the emotional reactions of the young men were more complex than the simple observations reported by Funkenstein and his colleagues. The determination of the subjects' predominant emotional coping style was just that—the predominant style. In many instances, men classified as having one predominant emotional coping style exhibited much of the emotional and behavioral characteristics of other styles. For example, it was not uncommon for a subject classified as Anger-Out to report having strong feelings of anxiety or blame himself (i.e., internalize the anger) for his reaction to the stressful situation, and then express intense feelings of dislike to the interviewer. Therefore, it appears that the experience and expression of anger in response to stressful events is a complex process that involves many emotions and a wider range of behaviors than we may sometimes be willing to consider in our research. I would go a bit further to say that the experience and expression of anger is probably determined to a great extent by gender, age, ethnicity (or race), degree of intoxication, as well as a number of other factors. Each of these factors may also be related to the degree that stress is mastered, the cognitive performance when under stress, and the intensity of other emotions such as anxiety and depression.

In the 1985 Detroit Study mentioned earlier, the relationship between anger coping styles and socio-ecological stress was examined within a sample of 1,000 (approximately 50-percent white and 50-percent black) residents of the city of Detroit.[22–25] Socio-ecological stress was measured by the degree of crime, juvenile delinquency, divorce, population density, residential mobility, and general dissatisfaction with the residential area in which respondents lived. Also included in the stress measure were the level of income and the employment status of individuals who took part in the study. Based on information derived from these factors and the census data for Detroit, Ernest Harburg and his associates were able to locate high and low stress areas that were inhabited primarily by white residents, and high and low socio-ecological stress areas where the residents were mostly black. Although Harburg examined several factors related to hypertension, for the time being I would draw your attention to the relationship between anger-coping styles and the degree of chronic environmental stress that is a permanent fixture of the day-to-day world in which these individuals reside.

Unlike the laboratory reactions obtained by Funkenstein and his associates at Harvard, the anger-coping styles identified in the Detroit Study were based on responses to several common social situations involving an unjustifiable provocation by authority figures (e.g., policemen, boss) or family members (e.g., spouse). All subjects were asked how they would handle their feelings of anger if they were verbally attacked and provoked. Several potential anger-coping responses were predetermined and committed to a questionnaire. Subjects indicated whether they would either get angry and keep the feeling to themselves (Anger-In Group), get angry and express the feeling (Anger-Out Group), or get angry but bypass it and focus on a problem-solving approach to the anger-provoking situation (Anger-Reflection Group). Curiously, in the relationship between these anger-coping styles and stress, the degree of environmental stress had no impact on the mode of anger expression. There was no difference in the number of subjects who were Anger-In, Anger-Out, or Anger-Reflection in the high- and low-stress living conditions. Some interesting differences did show up between men and women as well as between blacks and whites in their anger coping styles; but still, the degree of stress had no bearing on the manner in which anger was expressed. The differences between men and women and between blacks and whites will be discussed in the Chapter 6. In the meantime, there is an important finding from the National Survey of Black Americans that is relevant here.

It has been argued that the AHA! Syndrome plays a role in health problems because strong feelings of anger-hostility play a crucial role in generating life stress. To test this hypothesis, Clifford Broman and I examined the relationship between the degree of anger expression in response to personal distress in the past and to recent life stress, as exhibited in a nationally representative sample of 713 black adults who had answered the NSBA.[21] Life stress was measured by responses to four questions: Over the past month, have you had.family (or marriage, or money, or job.problems? Basically, four important findings emerged from this research. First, the frequency with which anger is expressed outwardly at people and objects in the environment may be an important predictor of negative life events for black Americans. In other words, those respondents with the highest level of Anger-Out experienced a greater number and degree of negative life events. Second, negative life events were associated with an increased number of health problems for black Americans in the NSBA. Third, is that the number of negative life events and the frequent outward expression of anger were independent predictors of health problems; and fourth, individuals with the highest level of anger were more emotionally disturbed. Therefore, anger may be a risk factor for health problems via two pathways: (1) by its association with negative and stressful life events, and (2) by itself. Our findings provide some evidence for the operation of these pathways. For example, the finding that anger conflict (Anger-Out) is associated with a greater number of stressful life events supports the perspective that people who have difficulty in handling their anger are more likely to destroy the important supportive relationships and networks with others that could otherwise buffer or mediate the connection between negative life events and health problems.

While there is a notable lack of research relating anger to life events, our findings are quite similar to those recently reported by Judy Siegel for white adolescents.[28] In her study, those adolescent males and females who scored higher on the anger-expression measure (Anger-Out) were more dissatisfied with their lives, had lower self-esteem, and experienced more negative life events. Although a bit speculative, these findings might indicate that talking about anger and expressing anger outwardly can intensify and prolong the experience of stressful life events.

It has been argued by theorists and researchers such as Carol Tavris,[29] Raymond Novaco,[30] and G.R. Patterson[31] that individuals who have problems managing their anger behave in ways which enhance angry and hostile interactions with others and generate more psychologic distress (e.g., increased levels of anxiety and depression; disturbed ability to concentrate) for themselves. Through negative and combative interpersonal behaviors, such persons may cause many unpleasant life events—job loss; divorce or marital difficulties; loss of friends and other avenues of social and emotional support—as well as engage in such negative health behaviors, as excessive cigarette smoking and drinking, overeating, or ignoring early symptoms of fatigue and ill health. These factors, in turn, may operate to increase their susceptibility to infectious diseases and health problems.

Returning to our findings from the NSBA—while data relevant to the first health-risk pathway show that anger style among blacks is a predictor of negative life events that in turn predict health problems—the data relevant to the second pathway show that anger expression is an independent predictor of health problems. As pointed out earlier, the maladaptive effects of anger in the etiology of psychoneurosis and depression have long been emphasized in clinical and experimental research concerned with the manifestation of personality disturbances. However, anger—particularly when manifested as chronic hostility—has recently been linked with Type-A behavior, coronary heart disease, malignant neoplasms, and death from all causes combined. Most contemporary theorists view the experience and expression of anger as one of several outcomes of a process initiated by certain frustrating and/or stressful external events, but it has been proposed further that the anger can be elicited by external events prior to cognitive assessment and interpretation.[31] Some investigators (Ernest Harburg[32], Raymond Novaco[33,33]) have argued that the individual's reconstruction of the external event (e.g., attributions about the intention of other persons) serves to elicit intense physiologic as well as emotional arousal; other researchers (Edwin Megargee,[34] James Averill[35]) believe that the experience and expression of anger may be best conceptualized as a "transactional response" to provocation, serving to regulate the emotional discomfort usually associated with stressful and problematic interpersonal relationships.

In either case, how might the experience and expression of anger account for increased health problems? First of all—as reviewed earlier—there is an abundance of evidence that, when cognitive appraisal of a situation results in a sense of danger and threat or a need for continuous mental efforts to cope with the situation, a characteristic defense-reaction or fight/flight pattern is observed. This pattern consists of an elevated blood pressure, increased pumping of blood by the heart along with shunting of blood to the skeletal muscles, and increased secretion of epinephrine, norepinephrine, and cortisol. Anger—which most researchers would define as an emotional state consisting of feelings of irritation, annoyance, fury, and rage and accompanied by heightened activation of the autonomic nervous system—may be one of the predominant emotional reactions that characterize the defensive reaction to stressful and unpleasant events.

Although this is somewhat speculative, individuals with high levels of anger conflict may experience an excess in neuroendocrine and cardiovascular response to stressful and provocative environmental demands—an excess that contributes to the pathogenesis of health problems. For example, if cortisol levels are increased during periods of anger conflict, this could potentiate both the metabolic and cardiovascular effects of catecholamines, which could in turn accelerate endothelial injury and lead to atherogenesis—as noted at the beginning of the chapter—by way of increased lipid mobilization. High levels of anger conflict associated with the defense-reaction pattern could also be related to depression of immune function (e.g., NK cell activity), where the end result would be a reduced ability to reject tumors.

There is a strong need for research to examine these relationships especially among black populations, whose members for the most part are confronted with a tremendous amount of chronic stress and racism. It is entirely feasible that anger-hostility could be related to the increased cancer mortality among blacks, as a function of the strained and problematic pattern of interactions between blacks and whites. The increased cancer mortality may also be a consequence of stressful and hostile interactions with important sources of social support such as family members, friends, and co-workers. This hypothesis is in line with the findings of Drs. Graves and Thomas that future cancer victims lack a close relationship with their parents and tend to have early human ties that are generally very disturbed and unsatisfactory.[7]

In any case, the relationship between stress and the AHA! Syndrome—although important in the link between emotions and disease—is not well researched. There does appear to be a strong thread of evidence in support of a relationship between the way anger is managed and the performance of individuals under stress. The findings from research on black Americans indicates an association between health problems and both high levels of anger expression and negative life events. However, due to the cross-sectional nature of these data, definitive statements cannot be made as to whether problems with anger expression and negative life events precede or are consequences of health problems for black Americans. Research to sort out the mechanisms whereby anger conflict and chronic stress are translated into disease processes is strongly needed. And this is especially true for black Americans, because of their substantially shorter life span.

3

Cardiovascular Disease
and the AHA! Syndrome

Medical literature has long suggested a link between personality factors and both essential hypertension and heart disease.[1-6] The most notable research in this area has been that relating anger–hostility (most often, suppressed anger–hostility) and aggression to essential hypertension, as well as the work relating the Type-A behavior pattern to ischemic heart disease.

Hypertension is one of the most frequently encountered disorders in medical practice and constitutes a significant risk factor for cardiovascular diseases such as stroke and myocardial infarction. Yet a recognizable specific cause (e.g., kidney disease, endocrine abnormalities, narrowing of the renal arteries) can be found in only 15 percent of patients with hypertension.[7,8] In approximately 85 percent of all hypertensive cases, therefore, the persistently elevated blood pressure cannot be attributed to any known organic cause and is referred to as "primary" or"essential" hypertension. Hypertensive blood-pressure readings are found in a large number of people and has been estimated that 40 million Americans show abnormal blood-pressure readings. Because of its frequency and its unknown etiology, as well as the complexity of its pathophysiology, essential hypertension has received more investigative attention than any other disease.

Among black Americans, the prevalence of essential hypertension is roughly twice that for whites. In addition, blacks are more likely to suffer from hypertensive vascular diseases. The reasons for this higher rate of hypertension morbidity and mortality in black adults are not presently known. In seeking an explanation, investigators have been giving increasing emphasis to the factors that initiate the disease as well as those that sustain it. Genetic or constitutional differences, abnormalities in the transport of sodium in red blood cells, increased sodium retention, dietary insufficiencies, psychological and personality factors, and psychosocial stresses have been particularly emphasized.

THE HYPERTENSIVE PERSONALITY

Studies of the psychological and personality characteristics of individuals with essential hypertension stem from the work of three pioneering researchers. In 1929, on the basis of his systematic study of the fight-or-flight response, Walter B. Cannon identified a complex adrenaline–mediated reaction involving increases in blood pressure, muscle tension, vasodilation, visceral vasoconstriction, and biochemical changes associated with energy mobilization.[9] Some years later, in 1947, Francis Dunbar made popular the notion that a specific personality type is associated with a particular psychosomatic disease.[1] Most pertinent to the present discussion is the psychoanalytically oriented work of Franz Alexander, who in 1939 proposed that hypertension results from a conflict between the desire to express hostility and the desire to be submissive and passive.[2,3] Alexander's ideas stimulated much of the modern–day research that has focused on the role of suppressed hostility in the personality of essential hypertensives. Alexander's work represents the most well-integrated hypothesis of the "hypertensive personality." Basically, Alexander proposed that hypertension arises from the inability of certain individuals to reconcile their needs for dependency and for expressing anger. According to Alexander.

> A very pronounced conflict between passive, dependent, feminine, receptive, tendencies and over-compensatory, competitive, aggressive hostile impulses which leads to fear and increases a flight from competition towards the passive dependent attitude. Characteristic for the hypertensive patient is, however, his inability to relieve freely either one of the opposing tendencies: neither can he freely accept one's passive dependent attitude nor truly express his hostile impulses. A kind of emotional paralysis can be observed which results from two opposing emotional attitudes blocking each other. The more they give in to their dependent compliant tendencies, the greater becomes their reactive hostility to those to whom they submit (Alexander, 1987, p. 148).[3]

Alexander and many of the other psychodynamically oriented investigators at the time thought that the inhibition of these hostile impulses contribute to elevated blood pressure by means of a generalized constriction of the arterioles throughout the vascular system. Furthermore, the intense and prolonged blood-pressure elevations involved in the chronic inhibition of hostility, and the high level of vascular resistance and anxiety associated with emotional conflict would ultimately result in the blood pressure becoming permanently elevated. In the case of hypertension, the increased vascular resistance was thought to be the result of an increase in vasomotor impulses to smooth muscles of the arteriole or perhaps of some circulating pressor substance such as norepinephrine. Support for Alexander's hypothesis was initially derived from his own clinical observations of hypertensive patients and the research of a close associate, L.J. Saul.[10] A host of other clinicians and psychosomatic researchers also reported that hypertensive patients—while often gentle, poised, and apparently easy-going—are actually filled with tightly restrained aggressive and hostile impulses.[11-14] Since these earliest psychodynamically oriented investigations, a large number of studies have reported a relationship between hypertension, anger, hostility, and aggression—using a wide variety of psychological questionnaires. In the remainder of this section I will summarize a few of the major studies that were conducted during the past 10 years.

The Detroit Study

As explained in Chapter 2, one of the purposes of the Detroit Study in the 1970s was to examine the relationship between anger-coping styles and chronic socio-ecological stress in a sample of 1,000 residents of the city of Detroit.[5-7,15] Another major aim of this study was to determine whether certain anger-coping styles are related to hypertension, and—if so—whether the degree of socio-ecological stress modifies the relationship between anger-coping style and hypertension. In other words, would blood pressure and the prevalence of hypertension be greater for subjects who had a suppressed-anger (Anger-In) coping style and who also resided in areas where there was a high level of stress. As expected, the results indicated that an Anger-In coping response is associated with higher diastolic blood pressure for both blacks and whites as well as for both males and females.

Although the level of blood pressure and the prevalence of hypertension was greater for blacks, males, and residents of high-stress neighborhoods, the relationship between anger-coping style and hypertension was essentially the same for all the gender and race groups making up the population. Results from the first report of the Detroit Study indicated that systolic and diastolic blood-pressure levels for black males living in high-stress areas were higher than those of any other groups. Of most importance was the finding that suppressed anger related significantly to elevated diastolic blood pressure for black males living in high-stress areas and white males living in low stress areas. Black men from the low stress areas with hypertension tended to keep their anger in and to deny feeling guilty, while white male residents of high stress areas who had hypertension felt guilty after expressing their anger. Overall, the percentage of diagnosed hypertension was 12.5 percent for respondents classified as using the Anger-Out coping style as compared to 19 percent for respondents using the Anger-In coping style.

The summary of findings for the female residents of Detroit showed that for black female residents of high-stress neighborhoods, an Anger-In coping response to provocations was again associated with hypertension. White female residents of low-stress areas who used the Anger-In coping response to provocations had higher blood pressures than their counterparts who expressed anger outwardly. Furthermore, there were no differences in blood pressure between black women with Anger-In and Anger-Out coping styles who resided in low-stress areas, or for white women with these coping styles who resided in the high-stress areas.

It is difficult to understand exactly what new knowledge Harburg gained about the role of stress and anger-coping styles in essential hypertension. Addressing this difficulty, psychologist W. Doyle Gentry reanalyzed the original data to examine more fully the effects of race, gender, socio-ecological stress, and habitual anger-coping styles on systolic and diastolic blood pressure and the risk of being classified as hypertensive. After adjusting for age and relative weight, the results indicated that: (1) blacks and all individuals with high levels of Anger-In had higher diastolic blood pressure; (2) blacks and all males had higher systolic blood pressure; (3) anger expression was inversely related to systolic blood pressure, but only for females; (4) all four factors (race, gender, stress, anger-coping style) were independently related to the relative risk of having hypertension, and (5) the odds of having hypertension were higher for blacks, males, persons with high suppressed anger (Anger-In) score and residents of high-stress areas. Most importantly, an individual's odds of having hypertension increased if he or she had more than one of the three risk factors. Of the individuals with no risk factors, 9 percent had hypertension, compared to a 33-percent hypertension rate for individuals with three risk factors.

The Tampa Study

The Tampa Study was directed by this author. Completed in 1984 as part of the requirement for my Ph.D., it represented an attempt to conduct a study similar to the Detroit Study.[16–18] Although the data reported by Ernest Harburg and W. Doyle Gentry remain quite impressive and indicate a relatively strong relationship between hypertension and suppressed hostility (Anger-In), it is quite possible that the adult subjects in the Detroit Study acquired their anger-coping styles as a reaction to having high blood pressure or being diagnosed as having hypertension. In other words, did the conflict about expressing anger precede the high blood pressure problem, or was it a reaction to being diagnosed as having hypertension? Therefore, a study using adolescents subjects, who had no prior history of hypertension, would provide strong evidence for the role of suppressed anger-hostility in elevated blood pressure.

The purpose of the Tampa Study, therefore, was to investigate the relationship between the prevalence of elevated blood pressure and several personality and traditional risk factors for hypertension in a sample of 603 white and 447 black adolescents (ages 15–17) who were enrolled in high-school health science courses in Tampa, Florida. All subjects had their blood pressure, weight, and height measured as part of the unit of study on cardiovascular disorders. Although a number of personality and traditional risk factors significantly predicted elevated blood pressure for both blacks and whites as well as for males and females, suppressed anger (Anger-In) turned out to be the most important predictor of elevated blood pressure for adolescents in the Tampa Study. Among blacks and whites, those who generally harbored grudges and suppressed their anger had higher systolic and diastolic blood pressure. Interestingly enough, familial factors—that is, whether the student's parents had hypertension or heart disease—were found to be independent predictors of blood pressure only for the white adolescents. So it seems that familial (or genetic) factors and other traditional risk factors such as weight were not particularly strong predictors of elevated blood pressure for black adolescents, but psychological measures of anger (particularly, suppressed anger) consistently predicted elevated blood pressure for black and white as well as male and female adolescents.

To gain a better understanding of the relationship between Anger-In and blood pressure, I divided the Tampa Study subjects into five subgroups based on their Anger-In scores. Figure 3-1 shows that the average systolic blood pressure for adolescent males and females was highest for those who had the highest anger-in scores. Although a similar pattern revealed itself for diastolic blood pressure, the relationship between Anger-In and systolic blood pressure was especially strong.

In a subsequent report of the Tampa Study data, I wanted to determine whether the relationship between emotional factors and blood pressure would be similar for adolescents who are more than 20-percent underweight, normal weight, and greater than 20-percent overweight for their age and height.[19] This inquiry was stimulated by the fact that weight had proven to be the second most important factor in the prediction of blood pressure. As expected, the blood pressure turned out to be highest among adolescents who were greater than 20 percent overweight. However, few of the other traditional risk factors were related to blood pressure for those adolescents who were greater than 20 percent overweight (see Table 3-1). In contrast, psychologic measures that assessed suppressed anger and the intensity of angry reaction were significantly associated with blood pressure for adolescents within each of the weight categories.

What happened next still sends a chill through my bones: I moved from sunny southern Tampa to that hazy northern place called Ann Arbor. It was COLD! During that first winter I could not figure out whether my blood pressure was elevated due to the stress of dealing with a new work

Figure 3-1
Systolic blood pressure in relation to Anger-In scores: Five Tampa Study subgroups

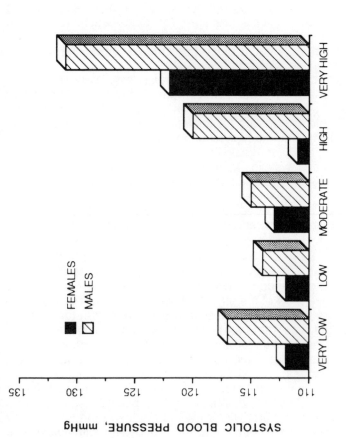

Source: Adapted from Johnson, E.H., Spielbergr, C. D., Worden, T. J., and Jacobs, G. Emotional and familial determinants of elevated blood pressure in black and white adolescent males. Journal of Psychosomatic Research 1987, 31:287–300; and Johnson, E.H., Schork, N., and Spielberger, C. D., Emotional and familial determinants of elevated blood pressure in black and white adolescent females. Journal of Psychosomatic Research 1987, 31:731–41.

Table 3-1

Blood Pressure in Relation to Weight, by Other Risk
and Emotional Variables: The Tampa Study

Variables	20% Underweight	Normal Weight	20% Overweight
Sex		++	
Race	++	+++	
Salt usage		+++	
Family history of hypertension		++	
Heart rate	++		
Anxiety	+++	+++	+++
Suppressed anger	+++	+++	+++

Note: ++ indicates the presence of a significant (p < .01) relationship and +++
indicates that the relationship was stronger (p < .001).

Source: Johnson, E.H. Interrelationship between psychological factors,
overweight, and blood pressure in adolescents. Journal of
Adolescent Health Care 1990, 11:310–318

environment, or whether this was indeed my own cardiovascular
fight/flight response alerting me that my frozen surroundings were a
threat to my very survival.

In any event, once I had settled in, my colleagues at the University
of Michigan and I conducted our first study of the relationship between
hypertension and anger.[20] We decided to see if anger and anxiety
would be related to elevated blood pressure outside of the clinic. One
reason for this decision was that average blood pressure outside of the
clinic has been shown to be a more important predictor of hypertensive
complications than blood pressure measurements taken in the
physician's office. In this study, we identified two groups of young adults
with mildly high (borderline hypertension) levels of blood pressure: one
group that had high blood pressure in the clinic and over the course of
seven days at home, and another whose blood pressure was elevated in

the clinic but was normal at home. Subjects in both groups completed the same measures of the experience and expression of anger and anxiety that I had used with the adolescent sample in Tampa. Our findings indicated that the group of borderline hypertensives who had high blood pressures at home over the course of seven days reported a greater intensity of anger, primarily in situations where they were pressured by time and deadlines. Also, they scored higher on the suppressed anger–hostility (Anger-In) measures than the borderline hypertensives whose average blood pressure returned to normal levels at home. Overall, the pattern of these findings indicated that individuals with elevated blood pressure across many situations—at the screening examinations, in the clinic, and at home—were psychologically different from the individuals whose blood pressure was elevated only at the initial screening examination.

In a recent and related study,[21] I examined the association between laboratory blood-pressure reactions to stress and blood pressure readings obtained at home for four weeks.[21] As expected, in the laboratory, subjects with hypertensive parents had higher blood pressure at rest and during exposure to stressful tasks than subjects with normotensive parents. The home blood pressure of the subjects with hypertensive parents was also higher over the 28 days, and these subjects scored higher on measures of anger and submissiveness. Of particular interest were results showing that the degree to which self-determined home blood pressure could be predicted was enhanced substantially by considering both the responses to stress and the individual's scores on the anger personality measures. Basically, a subject's response to laboratory stressors was predictive of the level of blood pressure measured 28 days following the laboratory examination. However, the accuracy of the prediction was substantially improved by considering the subject's scores on measures of the experience and expression of anger.

Michigan Statewide Blood Pressure Study

Data for the Michigan Statewide Blood Pressure Study were collected from 1980 to 1983 under the leadership of Drs. Victor Hawthorne and Bruce Brock, and the sample was selected to be representative of the adult population of the state of Michigan.[22] The present discussion, which focuses on the relationship between psychosocial factors and blood pressure, is based on the report prepared by Eric Cottington while at the Institute for Social Research at the University of Michigan. Of the 3,073 adults—aged 18–96 years—who participated in the baseline examination in 1980, a subsample of 444 subjects completed a special survey designed to assess more comprehensively a variety of psychosocial factors, including anger. What was discovered and reported by Cottington should come as no surprise.

Among both men and women in Michigan, those who generally did not express their emotions (including anger) and who tended to harbor grudges, hostility, and aggressive impulses had higher diastolic blood pressure. Among men, those with lower self-confidence and control over their lives had higher systolic and diastolic blood pressure, while those who reported poorer mental health had high diastolic blood pressure. Among women, those who rated their relationships with family members and best friends more poorly had higher systolic blood pressure.

One of the strengths of this study is the exclusion of physician-diagnosed hypertensives from the analyses. By taking multiple blood-pressure measurements at the subject's home, controlling for potential confounders, and using empirically derived measures of anger and other psychosocial factors, some of the limitations of previous studies were addressed. Therefore, the significant relationships observed between suppressed emotions (anger, specifically) and elevated blood pressure can not be explained away by the effects of a biased sample or risk factors for hypertension.

Occupational Stress, Suppressed Anger, and Hypertension in Pittsburgh

Surely, the driving force behind all these studies considered here is that being exposed to a stressful situation is not sufficient to cause disease. In fact, several research studies suggest that an individual does not feel the ill health effects of a particular stressor without being made vulnerable to them by some prior condition or circumstances—as in the case of the exaggerated cardiovascular response to stress observed among individuals with a parental history of hypertension. A better understanding of the relationship between health problems and stress should result from studies that not only measure exposure to stressful environmental events, but also determine how the individual generally copes with stress. In the case of hypertension, the suppressed anger coping style would be predicted to modify relationships between hypertension and stress. However, before looking into the modifying effects of suppressed anger I want to describe the findings of a few general studies on job stress and hypertension. In one of the most cited studies in this area, S. Cobb and R.M. Rose examined the prevalence of hypertension among 4,325 air traffic controllers.[23] Basically, they found that those controllers who worked in high density towers had a significantly greater prevalence of hypertension than those who worked in low density towers. Because density related to the amount of air traffic, Cobb and Rose inferred that differences in prevalence of hypertension might be explained by a difference in workload. And indeed a follow-up study among air traffic controllers revealed that individuals with new cases of hypertension had greater blood pressure elevations on days when there was a high workload.[24]

Another study had also examined this relationship between workload—as determined by job duties—and blood pressure. The subjects in this investigation were 148 employees of NASA—some of them intimately involved with the launching of a rocket to the moon, and some with no responsibility for the launch. Those involved in the launching were more educated and more likely to be employed as professionals, managers, or highly skilled technicians. It was assumed that the employees involved with the launch would have a greater workload and a higher level of responsibility. Interestingly enough, there was found no significant difference between the blood pressure levels of those who were involved with the launching and those who had no such responsibility. However, for other studies that assess the actual degree of job stress—rather than assume that job duties are a determination of workload—have provided support for the relationship between workstress and hypertension.[26–28] For example, a study by Jim House and his associates who monitored 353 workers in the rubber industry, revealed that workload, "intrinsic rewards" (i.e., utilization of skills), and role conflict were significantly associated with hypertension—even after controlling for variables such as obesity, age, and cigarette smoking.[29,30]

Certainly one of the most stressful work-related situations is the threat of job loss. To find out just how stressful, S.V. Kasl and S. Cobb were available in one such situation to study the relationship between job loss and elevated blood pressure among 150 married men of ages 35–60 who held a variety of blue-collar jobs.[31] These men, and a group of men who were not experiencing job loss, were followed for two years and given frequent blood-pressure examinations. The overall pattern of results from the study revealed that the men who were not experiencing job loss showed no significant long-term trends in blood pressure. Among those men experiencing job loss, however, their blood pressure levels during the anticipation of job loss and the actual unemployment were higher than during their later stabilization on new jobs. Unfortunately, information pertaining to anger-hostility coping styles were not measured in this most important study.

Although several studies do show a significant relationship between suppressed anger and hypertension, it should be possible further to test whether individuals who suppress anger and are also experiencing stressful situations that chronically provoke anger are at greater risk of hypertension than persons who are under less stress or persons who express their anger. This was precisely the catalyst behind the research conducted in the 1980s by Eric Cottington and his colleagues at the University of Pittsburgh.[32,33] More precisely, their research examined the modifying effect of suppressed anger on the relationship between hypertension and job stress among a random sample of male hourly workers, age 40–63 years. All of the men were employed at one of two manufacturing plants in the metropolitan

Pittsburgh area. Because of this sampling from two different plants, the study provided a unique opportunity to look for consistency in the modifying effects of suppressed anger across work places.

As hypothesized, hypertension was most strongly related to job stress among those men who chronically experienced but suppressed their anger. Specifically, the relationships between hypertension and both "job-future ambiguity" and "dissatisfaction with co-workers and promotions" were consistently modified by suppressed anger among the workers in both plants. And the prevalence of hypertension was highest for those men who experienced high levels of both job stress and suppressed anger. Furthermore, the modifying effect of suppressed anger on the relationship between hypertension and job stress was independent of the associations between known risk factors (e.g., age, weight, smoking, alcohol consumption, family history of hypertension) for hypertension. Overall, these results lend support to the notion that the etiologic relationship between stress and hypertension is a multifactorial one. Another way of looking at it is that the relationship between suppressed anger and hypertension is a multifactorial one.

Another team of researchers at the University of Pittsburgh—directed by psychologist Stephen Manuck—has directed its attention to understanding this multifactorial nature of the relationship between anger and hypertension.[34] Somewhat uniquely, their research attempts to establish how personality factors mediate the linkage between psychophysiologic responses to behavioral (or laboratory) stressors and essential hypertension. In other words, this approach is different because it would integrate the personality and psychophysiologic-response-to-stress approaches to hypertension research into a general model of idiosyncratic cardiovascular responses to stress.

According to one of the major premises of this research approach, the heightened autonomic reaction to stress that precedes the development of hypertension may conceivably originate in either hereditary or else psychological factors, or may reflect an interaction between both types of factors.[34,35] To test this hypothesis, healthy young adult males with and without a parental history of hypertension had their blood pressure levels and heart rates measured while they performed difficult mental arithmetic problems in the presence of the experimenter. In addition, the subjects' levels of anxiety and anger experienced before and during the difficult mental arithmetic task were measured. As has been noted in previous research, the sons of hypertensive parents had greater heart-rate and blood-pressure elevations during the math test, compared to the sons of parents without hypertension. Of most importance in the context of this discussion, the heart-rate stress response of persons with hypertensive and normotensive parents differed significantly only among those who experienced the greatest anxiety and anger when engaged in the stressful math task. On the other hand, the heart rate responsivity to stress was unrelated to the parents' history of hypertension among sons who reported little increase in anxiety or anger while performing the difficult arithmetic task. In other words, persons with a parental history of hypertension have a stronger potential to exhibit higher cardiovascular responses to mental stress—a potential that is apparently to be proportional to the degree of negative affect experienced before and during stressful tasks.

Another approach to understanding the role of psychological factors in hypertension involves the determination of assertiveness deficits—an important indicator of interpersonal skills and social competence.[36,37] The rationale behind this approach is that the strong tendency of hypertensives to suppress anger and hostility may mean they cannot effectively assert themselves and express feelings. Although the usual approach is to determine the range of assertiveness from the subject's response to a questionnaire, direct observation offers an opportunity to assess social competence even more precisely. If hypertensive patients do have problems expressing their anger, it is possible that they may be unaware of, and unable to report on, their assertiveness and social-skills deficit. Fortunately, the research group at the University of Pittsburgh has developed a laboratory role-play test of assertiveness to investigate the function of interpersonal deficits in hypertension.[34] The typical role-play situation involves a staged interaction between the subject, who is often seated in an interviewing room, and an experiment-team confederate whose function is to prompt the subject and increase the difficulty of the interaction. In this setting, a narrator describes an interpersonal situation that requires assertive responses (e.g., someone enters a line directly in front of you). The confederate initiates the interaction, and the subject is instructed to respond as if he or she were actually experiencing the situation. Meanwhile, blood pressure, heart rate, and other psychophysiologic data are gathered. In most cases, the role-play is videotaped for later scoring.

Whereas a number of important findings regarding the validity of the assertiveness role-play situation have been uncovered by the research group at Pittsburgh, the relationships between subjects' psychophysiologic responsivity and assertiveness are of most interest. Basically, their results have revealed that there is no reliable association between blood pressure changes during the role-play and assertiveness in subjects with normal blood pressure. However, among hypertensives, positive correlations were found—indicating that heightened physiologic reactivity is associated with greater, not less, assertiveness. Several interesting findings emerged when the group of hypertensives were subdivided into those who had the greatest systolic blood pressure elevations during the role-play (Group 1) versus those whose systolic blood pressure was largely attenuated (Group 2). For example, hypertensive subjects in Group 1 were found to be significantly more assertive than hypertensives in Group 2 and equal in assertiveness to subjects with normal blood pressure levels. Of most importance are the findings which showed that hypertensives in Group 1 differed from normotensives in verbal content and expressive mannerisms which are behavioral categories indicative of greater hostility and aggressiveness.

Hostility, Sympathetic Nervous System Activity, and Hypertension

One of the characteristic features of the early stage of essential hypertension is sympathetic nervous system overactivity as reflected by a high plasma concentration of norepinephrine.[38,39] Plasma renin activity is also elevated in some patients with essential hypertension; and since the sympathetic nervous system plays an important role in regulating renin release by the kidney, it is possible that an elevated plasma renin activity in hypertension could be a marker indicating a generalized increase in cardiovascular and sympathetic nervous system overactivity.[40] To find out, Murray Esler (a visiting research scientist from the Baker Medical Research Institute located in Victoria State, Australia) directed a study in 1977 at the University of Michigan Medical Center's Division of Hypertension to determine whether elevated plasma renin activity is indeed an expression of sympathetic nervous system overactivity.[41] The study compared indexes of sympathetic activity in 16 hypertensive patients with high plasma renin levels, 15 hypertensive patients with normal plasma renin activity, and 20 patients with normal blood pressure and normal plasma renin activity. Esler discovered that the hypertensive patients with elevated plasma renin activity exhibited a high level of plasma norepinephrine, thus verifying the hypothesized connection.

In an effort to ascertain the possible origins of sympathetic nervous system overactivity, the subjects in this study were then subjected to some rather sophisticated pharmacologic manipulations to lower or suppress the plasma renin activity level. Interestingly enough, the pharmacologic manipulations lowered the plasma renin activity level, but the level of plasma norepinephrine (and therefore the sympathetic activation) remained elevated. Psychological factors were also investigated as having a role in the generation of sympathetic nervous system overactivity.[41,42] In the hypertensive patients, anxiety levels were found to be normal, however; suppressed hostility was a prominent feature in hypertensive patients, but only in those with elevated plasma renin activity. Overall, the hypertensive patients with high levels of plasma renin were controlled, guilt prone, and submissive, with a high level of unexpressed anger. The research team concluded that the pathogenesis of the blood pressure elevation in the patients with elevated plasma renin activity may involve suppression of hostility as a persistent reaction pattern, leading to chronic activation of the sympathetic nervous system.

The research by Esler stimulated another study that was carried out by Patrick Sullivan under the leadership of Vincent DeQuattro at the University of Southern California School of Medicine in Los Angeles County.[43] Vincent DeQuattro had worked on the research project with Murray Esler, and both men were medical doctors—not psychologists. In fact, when I joined the Division of Hypertension at the University of Michigan in 1985 I became the first psychologist to follow up the research leads that had been uncovered by Esler and DeQuattro.

Be that as it may, the study by Patrick Sullivan in 1981 was conducted to determine whether basal (resting) blood pressure or blood pressure response to stress is related to sympathetic nervous system activity or to psychological measures of suppressed anger, anxiety, and depression. A total of 15 hypertensive patients and 13 individuals with normal blood pressure were compared on the psychological measures and their blood-pressure, heart-rate, and plasma norepinephrine and epinephrine responses to an isometric handgrip exercise and a mental-challenge stress task consisting of a serial subtraction problem. As expected, a greater number of the hypertensive patients had higher levels of suppressed anger and scored higher on the anxiety and depression measures than the normal control subjects. Before exposure to the mental challenge stress, the value readings for plasma norepinephrine and blood pressure were greater in hypertensives. During the tasks, however, the increase in norepinephrine, blood pressure, and heart rate was similar for both the hypertensive and normal blood pressure groups. The investigators concluded that hypertensives have an increased neurogenic, or sympathetic, tone related perhaps to inward anger and anxiety and that suppressed anger—via this increased basal neurogenic tone—may be the pathogenic factor in some patients with primary or essential hypertension.

In yet another study, conducted in Switzerland, a team of researchers directed by Charles Perini and working under the leadership of Fritz Buhler also discovered a relationship between suppressed aggression and noradrenaline, or norepinephrine, activity.[44] The study examined the effects of suppressed aggression on the reactivity of the sympathetic nervous and cardiovascular systems in two groups of 24 subjects (age 18–24 years), each with either borderline hypertension or normal blood pressure and no family history of hypertension. As with the previous study reported by DeQuattro, Sullivan, and their associates, responses of blood pressure, heart rate, and plasma norepinephrine were measured before and during the application of a mental-challenge stress task. There were a number of interesting findings. For one thing, borderline hypertensive subjects with suppressed aggression had significantly higher heart rates and diastolic blood pressure and a greater noradrenaline reactivity to mental stress than the borderline hypertensive subjects without suppressed aggression and the subjects with normal blood pressure. The team of investigators concluded that suppressed aggression is responsible for the observed increase in sympathetic nervous system activity, heart rate, and diastolic blood pressure during stress, and also that suppressed aggression may be a determinant in the development of a more severe hyperadrenergic form of hypertension.

The notion that hypertensive individuals respond to laboratory stressors with greater elevations in blood pressure and heart rate than normotensives has become a controversial issue among those of us involved in hypertension research. For the most part, the hyperreactivity to mental stress appears to precede the development of hypertension, since such hyperreactivity is also found in normotensive offspring (children, adolescents, and adults) of parents with hypertension. Although numerous investigations conducted over the past 30 years have shown an association between elevated cardiovascular reactions to stress and familial factors, one of the major difficulties is that the pattern of cardiovascular responses tends to differ from study to study. Isolated systolic blood pressure elevations, isolated heart-rate reactions to stress, or a combined heart rate–blood pressure hyperreactivity to stress have been revealed in many studies. The problem remains that the physiological basis and significance of these differences in the pattern of cardiovascular responsiveness to stress are not yet understood.[45,46]

Despite the number of problems inherent to these studies, the importance of such research becomes apparent when one considers that the causes of hypertension are unknown in more than 80 percent of hypertensive patients, and that medical scientists have not been successful in predicting which individuals will develop hypertension. A multi-disciplinary approach to understanding these issues is currently under way, and one of the most powerful examples of this approach is the work of Dr. Bonita Falkner.[47,48] In Falkner study, adolescents with mild (i.e. borderline) hypertension were followed for five years after the initial measurements. Those who progressed from borderline to sustained hypertension exhibited a higher and more exaggerated cardiovascular response to mental stress and had a family history of hypertension. There is still a great deal of controversy over whether the hyperreactivity to mental stress constitutes a marker of some as yet unexplained pathophysiological mechanism (e.g., retention of sodium during stress) whereby the stress leads to hypertension. However, findings that show the blood pressure levels associated with natural stress (such as at work) to be more strongly related to organ damage (e.g., damage to peripheral vessels; hypertrophy of the left ventricle of the heart) than non–work related blood pressures serve to underscore the complexity of the relationship between stress and hypertension. Moreover, the issues are made more complex by the natural history of hypertension, which is not a static disease. In other words, the mechanisms responsible for blood pressure elevations may change as the disease continues to evolve.[46]

Emotional States and Blood Pressure in the Natural Environment

Despite the wealth of information about the relationship between psychological factors such as the AHA! Syndrome and hypertension, little is known about the relationship between blood pressure and emotional states of individuals as they ambulate in their natural environment. To a certain extent, this paucity of information reflects the technical difficulties inherent in obtaining reliable blood-pressure readings outside of the research laboratory or the hypertension treatment clinic. Another—and connected—reason for the lack of information in this area is that the taking of blood pressure measurements in the physician's office, using a sphygmomanometer, is considered to be the gold standard for diagnosing hypertension. However, in reality, blood pressure is constantly changing—subject to a variety of both psychological and physiological factors. Posture and exercise alter blood pressure—as do anger, anxiety, depression, and other strongly felt emotions. Overall, office measurements may vary so widely from the patient's norm that they provide an unreliable index for diagnosis and management of hypertension.[8]

During the past decade, ambulatory blood pressure monitoring (ABPM) units have been rigorously evaluated for clinical utility in the management of hypertensive patients. The key clinical premise for assessing ambulatory blood pressure is that repeated measurements taken over time provide a more valid estimate of average blood pressure than does a single reading.[49–54] In fact, several lines of evidence suggest that ABPM data constitute the better indicator of risk. First, clinic measurements may not accurately reflect the average 24-hour blood pressure. Second, several studies demonstrate convincingly that target organ damage correlates more closely to ambulatory blood pressure readings than to clinic measurements.[56,57] Third and finally, results of a few prospective investigations suggest that ambulatory blood pressure levels are better predictors of morbid events than are those measured in the clinic.[56]

ABPM provides a unique opportunity to study the relationship between blood pressure and psychological variables during daily activities. Although there is good evidence that elements of the AHA! Syndrome are related to elevated blood pressure and hypertension, most of the studies up until now, have relied on questionnaire measures of the psychological or emotional states and one or more blood pressure readings taken in a clinic or screening setting.

A study conducted by M. Sokolow and his associates is often

Figure 3-2
Average systolic blood pressure for moods, adjusted for individual differences in mean blood pressure

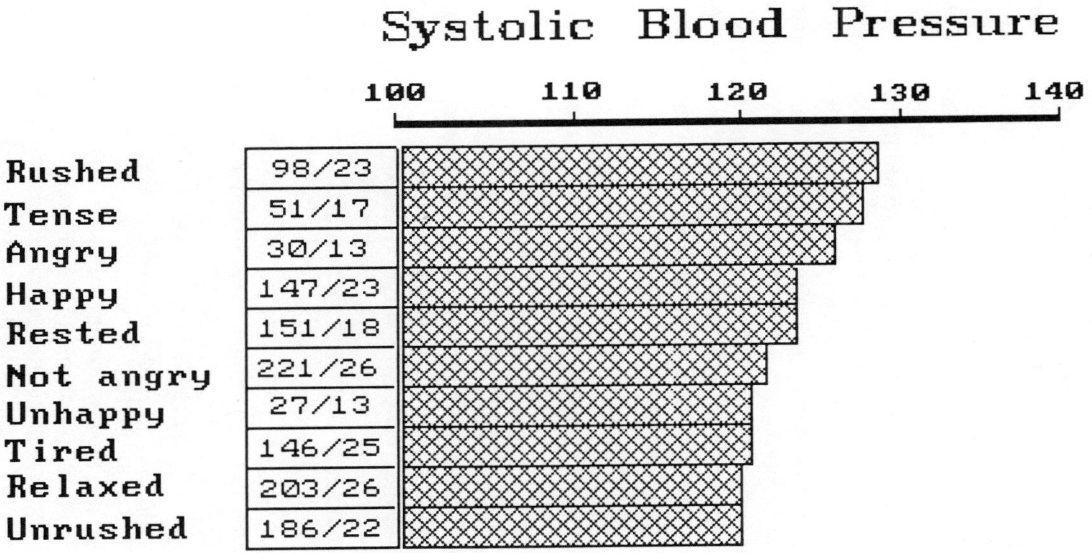

Systolic Blood Pressure

Mood	Value
Rushed	98/23
Tense	51/17
Angry	30/13
Happy	147/23
Rested	151/18
Not angry	221/26
Unhappy	27/13
Tired	146/25
Relaxed	203/26
Unrushed	186/22

Scale: 100 110 120 130 140

Source: Van Egeren, L.F. and Madarasmi, S., A computer-assisted diary (CAD) for ambulatory blood pressure monitoring. Reprinted with permission from <u>American Journal of Hypertension</u> 1988, 1;185S.

cited as one of the earliest to investigate the everyday covariation of emotional or psychological states and blood pressure.[49,50] In this study, 50 untreated hypertensives underwent ABPM at half-hour intervals over a two-day period. The emotional ratings form included 30 adjectives describing hostility, anxiety, alertness, depression, time pressures, and contentment. A negative-emotion scale was derived from the hostility, depression, anxiety, and time-pressure ratings. Sokolow and his associates found a significant relationship between elevated blood pressure and negative affect states during ordinary daily life. Moreover, this finding supported the hypothesis that individuals who view life situations as stressful and have occasions for negative emotional responses are the more likely to have elevated blood pressure.

Over the past decade a number of other excellent studies of hypertensive patients and normotensive controls have revealed that the perception of the environment as demanding and the occurrence of negative emotional states (hostility, anger, depression) are indeed related to ambulatory blood pressure readings. A recent study by Lawrence Van Egeren and Suthep Madarasmi is one good example.[54] In their study, the average 24-hour blood pressure of 16 male and 16 female employees of Michigan State University were monitored during a workday. The employees were primarily administrators, program managers, laboratory technicians, and secretaries. As shown in Figure 3-2, systolic blood pressure was highest when employees reported feeling rushed, tense, and angry. Feeling relaxed and unrushed was associated with the lowest systolic blood pressure.

LETHAL TYPE-A BEHAVIOR, CORONARY HEART DISEASE, AND THE AHA! SYNDROME

Despite considerable advances in medical research over the past 50 years, cardiovascular disease—and in particular, coronary heart disease (CHD)—remains the primary cause of early death in the United States. The terms "coronary heart disease," "atherosclerotic heart disease," and "ischemic heart disease" are often used interchangeably to refer to cardiac disease that leads to myocardial infarction or ischemia. In a general sense, CHD refers to a condition in which atherosclerosis is the primary cause of the coronary artery disease.[57,58] Indeed, the underlying condition in most cases of myocardial infarction, angina pectoris (ischemic pain), and sudden death is atherosclerosis—the accumulation of fatty deposits in the linings of the arteries. As indicated in Chapter 2, one of the major theories of the cause of atherosclerosis suggests that the sequence of events would involve: (1) endothelial damage—that is, to the inner lining of the artery—resulting from hemodynamic stress (increased blood pressure; turbulent blood flow around branching points of arteries) or circulating chemicals (for example, the stress-related catecholamines known as norepinephrine and epinephrine); (2) proliferation of arterial smooth-muscle cells in response to the injury; and (3) accumulation of lipoproteins and other cells causing plaques at the site of the injury.

Although acute clinical events presumably result from the occlusion of blood flow to the heart muscle, many instances of sudden death may be preceded by ventricular arrhythmia in response to some immediate stress. A large body of research has identified a set of risk factors (elevated serum cholesterol, hypertension, smoking, physical inactivity, age, gender, obesity, diabetes mellitus, and familial history) that are associated with CHD. However, even the best studies on the combining of these risk factors fail to identify most new cases of CHD. In fact, the so-called risk factors account for only about 50 percent of the incidence of CHD in middle-aged men in the United States.[58,60] Thus, Ansel Keys and other researchers maintain that the traditional risk factors do not perfectly predict the incidence of CHD or any other major health problems, for that matter.[59–62] It seems obvious that other factors are involved in the development of CHD.

One of the first psychosocial factors that was believed to play an important role in the development of CHD is referred to as the "Type-A behavior pattern" (TABP).[61] Interestingly enough, the modern-day description of the TABP is quite similar to the type of individual susceptible to CHD that was outlined by William Osler in 1892.[63] The future CHD candidate was described by Osler as "not the delicate, neurotic person but the robust, the vigorous in mind and body, the keen and ambitious man, the indicator of whose engine is always at full speed ahead." Some years later—in 1936—the Menningers studied patients with CHD and discovered that they were frequently characterized by a strong aggressive and hostile personality.[64] Frances Dunbar, one of the pioneers of psychosomatic medicine, went even further in 1943 by proclaiming that the aggressive, hard-driving, competitive, often hostile, and goal-directed behavior of CHD patients constitutes a coronary personality.

During those early years, a number of other psychosomatic-oriented psychiatrists confirmed the perception of the CHD patient as being overly aggressive and compulsively striving to achieve goals in as little time as possible. However, it was the work of cardiologists Ray Rosenman and Meyer Friedman in the 1960s and 1970s that convincingly demonstrated a link between CHD and the habits of behavioral and emotional response to daily life.[61,65] Rosenman and Friedman receive the credit not only for the name currently in use—the Type-A behavior pattern—but also for making the TABP an essential part of research in epidemiology and the treatment of CHD. This important scientific advancement hinged on their development of a structured and highly reliable interview for diagnosing TABP, along with demonstrating that the information derived from their interview could be used to predict future CHD. Then, however, a small investigation of the dietary habits of wives and husbands from the San Francisco Junior League convinced them that they were on the right track.

The dietary intake of cholesterol was identical for each couple, but yet the husbands' rate of CHD was substantially higher. Why this greater incidence of CHD among the husbands? It was the president of the Junior League who suggested that stress at work was probably contributing to the husbands' CHD. In order to investigate this factor then, Rosenman and Friedman mailed out questionnaires to 150 businessmen in the San Francisco community, asking respondents to indicate what habits they believed had contributed to heart attacks among their friends. Surprisingly, less than 5 percent reported that the friends' heart attacks were caused by excessive ingestion of fatty foods high in cholesterol, smoking cigarettes, or physical inactivity. On the other hand, approximately 70 percent of these businessmen indicated that excessive competitive drive, having to meet deadlines, and overindulgence were the most notable features of their friends who had heart attacks.

Although many different reasons have been advanced for Friedman and Rosenman's shift to the study of personality and behavioral factors in the etiology of heart disease, the one that I like best is the story about the furniture upholsterer who was summoned to reupholster the chairs in their waiting room. After going about his work for awhile, the man questioned the two cardiologists about their line of business because, he noted only a few inches at the edge of every chair was worn down.

Having had occasion to enjoy many visits with Ray Rosenman, I know that there are also a number of other reasons behind his quest for identification of the coronary-prone behavior pattern. In their 1974 book Type-A Behavior and Your Heart, Friedman and Rosenman describe the Type-A pattern as:

> an action-emotion complex that can be observed in any person who is aggressively involved in a chronic, incessant struggle to achieve more and more in less and less time, and if required to do so against the opposing efforts of other things or other persons. It is not psychosis or complex of worries or fears or phobias or obsessions, but a socially acceptable—indeed often praised—form of conflict. Persons possessing this pattern also are quite prone to exhibit a free-flowing but extraordinarily well-rationalized hostility. As might be expected, there are degrees in the intensity of this behavior pattern. Moreover, because the pattern represents the reaction that takes place when particular personality traits of an afflicted individual are challenged or aroused by a specific environmental agent, the results of this reaction (that is, the behavior pattern itself) may not be felt or exhibited by him if he happens to be in or confronted by an

environment that presents no challenge. For example, a usually hard-driving, competitive, aggressive editor of an urban newspaper, if hospitalized with a trivial illness, may not exhibit a single sign of Type-A behavior pattern. In short, for Type-A behavior pattern to explode into being, the environmental challenge must always serve as the fuse for this explosion. (Friedman and Rosenman, 1974, p. 84)[61]

In 1960, along with a number of collaborators, Friedman and Rosenman initiated a prospective epidemiological investigation referred to as the Western Collaborative Group Study (WCGS).[65,66] This study investigated the incidence of CHD in 3,154 men who were from 39 to 59 years old at the start of the study and were employed by ten California companies. A comprehensive set of data was obtained at the start-up and then each year until the WCGS was terminated 8.5 years later. The data included Type-A behavior, medical history for CHD and diabetes, total cholesterol, fasting triglycerides, beta/alpha lipoprotein ratio, blood pressure, smoking habits, exercise habits, education level, and annual income level. Death occurred in 140 men over the follow-up period—31 of their initial CHD event; 19 of a recurring CHD event; and 90 of non-CHD causes—while CHD developed in 257 subjects.

The findings of the WCGS indicated that the relative risk—that is, the probability of the disease occurring in a population exposed to the suspected factor—in males age 39–49 was 2.21 before adjustments for all other factors, and 1.97 after adjustment. For males 50–59, the relative risk ratio was 2.31 before adjustment and 1.98 after adjustment. Clearly the WCGS showed—for the first time in a thorough prospective study—that those men rated as having a Type-A behavior–emotional pattern at the onset of this study were twice as likely to develop CHD over the 8.5 years compared to men rated as Type-B (the opposite of Type-A). Moreover, the TABP was found to be a particularly good predictor of subsequent reinfarction. In addition to these findings, data from three separate research groups found that patients with Type-A behavior had more extensive coronary occlusion at the time of a diagnostic cardiac catheterization than their Type-B counterparts. Furthermore, two of these studies showed that the relationship between Type-A behavior and the degree of coronary artery disease persisted after taking into consideration other traditional risk factors.

In another well-known study—the Framingham Heart Study—1,674 men and women of age 45–77 years and free of CHD, were intensely examined between 1965 and 1967, and then reexamined eight years later.[60,61] Unlike the WCGS, both men and women participated in the Framingham Heart Study; and most importantly, Type-A behavior scores were derived from responses to a 300-item questionnaire, rather than from the structured interview. In addition to the Type-A behavior measure, the team of researchers derived measures reflective of the reactions to anger, situational stress, somatic strain, and psychosocial immobility. The anger scale measured ways of expressing and coping with anger (Anger-In, Anger-Out, anger-discuss; talking with a friend or relative). The situational stress scale measured situations in marriage, job, or life that would pose potential threats to the individual— such as nonsupport from the boss, job overload, and marital dissatisfaction. The somatic strain scale provided an index of physiological or behavioral responses indicative of stress, including anxiety and anger symptoms. Occupational mobility was indicated by changes in job or line of work and number of times promoted over the previous 10 years. The major findings linking these factors to CHD were published under the leadership of Drs. Susan Haynes and Saul Levine in 1978.[60] It was discovered that people who developed CHD over the follow-up period had scored higher on the initial Type-A questionnaire and were more likely to suppress their anger and hostility than their counterparts who remained free of heart disease. The gender differences revealed that women, of age 45–64, who developed CHD were higher in Type-A, suppressed hostility, anxiety and tension. For males aged 45 to 64, Type-A behavior was associated with a two-times greater risk of CHD, angina, and myocardial infarction when compared to Type-B men.

As a result of the findings from these and other studies, an independent review panel in 1981 recognized Type-A behavior as a risk factor for coronary artery disease.[67] Unfortunately—as Joel Dimsdale pointed out in a January 14, 1988 editorial in the New England Journal of Medicine—the "road has been a rocky one ever since, with a disturbingly high number of contradictory findings regarding the hypothesized dangers of this risk factor."[68]

Although a number of groups have attempted to replicate the WCGS findings, their results have been inconsistent.[69–72] Exceptionally strong criticisms about the relationship between Type-A behavior and CHD were voiced after a 1988 review and extension of the original WCGS database. As Joel Dimsdale indicated in his editorial, the recent findings "cast a long shadow indeed on the evidence supporting Type-A behavior as a risk factor." The review in question was prepared by Drs. David Ragland and Richard Brand, both with the School of Public Health at the University of California at Berkeley.[73] Basically, they studied the survival of the 257 male patients who had developed CHD at the 8.5-year phase of the WCGS. The results indicated that Type-A was unrelated to mortality among 26 men who died within 24 hours of a coronary event. However, of the 231 men who survived for 24 hours, the mortality rate associated with CHD among 160 Type-A men studied during 13 years was 19 per 1,000 compared to 32 among the 71 Type-B men who were followed for 11.5 years. In a nutshell, Ragland and Brand found that subsequent coronary mortality in men who suffered a first coronary event was unexpectedly lower among Type-As than Type-Bs.

At first glance, there appears to be little validity to the Type-A construct. But hold on a minute. Let's take a deeper look at the relationship between CHD and the components of Type-A behavior. In relying on the broad label of "Type-A behavior," it is possible that the core of the coronary-prone personality has not been adequately investigated. As it turns out, in 1977 psychologist Karen Mathews along with David Glass, Ray Rosenman, and Raymond Bortner reported findings after some analyses of the WCGS.[74] Their results showed that four of the seven Type-A interview items that discriminated between men with CHD and men free of CHD were related to anger and hostility dimensions of the AHA! Syndrome. In fact, two of the four items were actually self-reports of anger, and the response to these items was an acknowledgment that the men became angry more than once a week and that their of anger was often directed outwardly (Anger-Out) at other people. The remaining two items were based on ratings of "potential for hostility" and "explosive voice modulation" derived from the audio recording of the interview. And another reanalysis of the WCGS data, conducted by Margaret Chesney and her associates in the early 1980s, also showed that potential for hostility was the strongest component of Type-A behavior predicting subsequent coronary events.[75]

In 1985 psychologist Theodore (Ted) Dembroski reported on his component analysis of the Type-A interviews of patients who had undergone angiographic evaluation at Duke University Medical Center.[76] The purpose of this study was to determine whether the various measures of the components of Type-A are significantly related to incidences of coronary heart disease (total coronary index rating; number of coronary vessels occluded; history of angina; number of previous myocardial infarctions). A total of 131 patients (98 men and 33 women) were selected from a larger population of 2,000 patients who underwent diagnostic coronary angiography during the period from May 1976 to December 1981. Dembroski used a random sampling technique such that there were equal numbers of patients having 0–,2–, and 3– coronary vessel disease.

This study showed no relationship between Type-A behavior and the extent of CHD. However, potential for hostility and suppressed anger (Anger-In) were significantly and positively associated with disease severity, including history of angina and number of myocardial infarctions. Potential for hostility was measured by evaluating a subject's response to the Type-A interview questions involving a variety of frustrating circumstances in daily life (e.g., driving behind a slow-moving car; being kept waiting for an appointment; experiencing aggravation in the work place). Verbal responses indicative of harsh generalizations, usage of obscenities and the subjects' manners during the interview were evaluated for argumentative style and rudeness, as well as less overt forms of hostility such as condescension. The Anger-In, or suppressed-anger measure, was operationally defined by an "unwillingness in a variety of circumstances to overtly express frustration-induced hostility and/or anger." Although the Anger-In dimension was deduced to be independent of hostility, further analysis revealed a positive relationship between hostility and CHD indexes only in those patients who were rated high in suppressed anger. In other words, hostility and Anger-In were interactive in their relationship with CHD severity to the extent that the level of hostility was unrelated to coronary heart disease in those patients who openly expressed anger outwardly against the source of frustration.

Based on these findings, I have to agree with Joel Dimsdale that "it would be interesting to examine the data-set used by Ragland and Brand to learn whether the potential for hostility was related to long-term survival."[68] It would be equally interesting to determine if the other components of the AHA! Syndrome are predictive of long-term survival in men who participated in the WCGS. I am hopeful that this question will be addressed in future reports.

Another approach to studying the relationship between anger–hostility and Type-A behavior involves comparison of the psychophysiological responses of Type-A and Type-B subjects to stressful and challenging laboratory tasks.[77,78] For example, in 1978 and 1979 Ted Dembroski and his associates discovered that potential for hostility was most strongly related to systolic blood pressure and heart rate increases in response to stressful and challenging tasks. Interestingly enough, the Type-A subjects with high levels of hostility reacted to both high- and low-challenge conditions with heightened cardiovascular (i.e., blood pressure) reactivity. A few years later—in 1984—Eric Diamond and his associates at the University of Florida also discovered that Type-A subjects who had high levels of hostility and outwardly expressed anger exhibited the highest levels of physiological reactivity when harassed by a study-team confederate (who was making derogatory remarks about their performance).[79]

As indicated earlier, there is ample evidence of a stress-related hypersympathetic state in the early phase (mild or borderline) of essential hypertension. Whereas there is a similar body of research demonstrating that individuals with the Type-A behavior pattern exhibit hyperreactive responses to mental stress, the exact pathogenic mechanisms linking Type-A or hostility to coronary heart disease are not well understood.[4] Also, there are the problems related to demonstrating the independent relationship between a single variable (such as Type-A) and the health condition (in this case, CHD). In the process, important information about the relationships between the variable of interest and other risk factors that might contribute to the health condition are overlooked. Fortunately, several studies do shed light on this issue by examining the role of hostility and Type-A behavior in the elevation of other coronary risk factors such as alcohol consumption and cholesterol.

One important study in this area was reported by Carlos Camargo and associates[82] working at Stanford University.[80] The relationship between TABP and alcohol intake was investigated within a sample of 81 sedentary, but healthy, middle-aged (30–55 years of age) men. The men in the Type-A category reported drinking approximately twice as much alcohol as their non–Type-A counterparts. More specifically, the Type-A participants consumed 21.7 grams of ethanol per day, compared to 9.4 grams per day for the non–Type-A subjects. Furthermore, the relationship between alcohol consumption and Type-A behavior was not confounded by factors such as differences in income level or years of formal education or whether the men were cigarette smokers. For the most part, these result of this study are compatible with earlier studies of middle-aged men and premenopausal women, in which Type-A subjects were reported as drinking 1.2–2.2 times more than their Type-B counterparts.

Although the exact nature of the association between alcohol intake and the Type-A behavior pattern is unclear, it is highly possible that Type-As and highly hostile individuals may consume more alcohol (than Type-Bs or persons with low hostility) in an attempt to relax and get away from stress. On the other hand, the high consumption of alcohol may enhance the hostility and feelings of anger that characterize the Type-A. It is also possible that the higher intake of alcohol among Type-As may be partly related to job-demands differences. For example, previous research has revealed that Type-A behavior is related to long work hours and high occupational mobility, as well as nonsupportive job related interactions—the types of activities that result in co-workers talking about work-related problems over a drink.

EMOTIONS AND CHOLESTEROL

Elevated levels of total and low-density lipoprotein (LDL) cholesterol have been clearly recognized as one of the important risk factors for coronary artery disease in adults. The relationship between emotions and cholesterol is beginning to receive attention from researchers and the general public.[81–89] Most people in the United States are aware of the link between heart disease and high cholesterol, but only recently has research shown strong indications that personality and emotions contribute to the rise in cholesterol levels. For example, a study reported in 1987 by Gerdi Weidner and associates is an excellent example of the research needed in order to examine the combined or added contribution of the two classes of variables—psychological and physiological—in the stress–disease process.[81] The Weidner study was designed to examine the relationship of hostility and Type-A behavior to plasma lipids (specifically, cholesterol) and lipoproteins in a community sample of 352 women and men who were participants in the Family Heart Study conducted in Portland, Oregon. There were 182 women and 170 men included in the initial study and at the follow-up after a year; and the average age was 36, ranging from 16 to 69 years. Overall, the pattern of results from the initial study suggests that high levels of hostility among persons with a strong TABP is related to increased or elevated levels of plasma total and low-density-lipoprotein (LDL) cholesterol in both women and men. To a certain extent, the results obtained one year after the initial examination followed a similar pattern. Therefore, hostility among Type-As may contribute to the atherosclerotic process by keeping plasma total and LDL (the bad type) cholesterol elevated. It is conceivable, for example, that the hostile Type-A individual experiences more frequent feelings of anger and high-arousal stress situations, which increases the release of catecholamines as a result of sympathetic nervous system activation. In the long run, the excessive release of catecholamines might contribute to lipid mobilization and atherosclerosis. Confirmation of this scenario must come from future studies, however.

In another recent study, psychologist Ray Niaura and his colleagues at the Miriam Hospital in Providence, Rhode Island, investigated the relationship between cholesterol and psychological measures of defensiveness and repression.[85] The study evaluated personality types and cholesterol (total cholesterol; HDL cholesterol) and triglyceride levels among 42 men and 72 women. Niaura found that HDL and triglyceride levels did not differ according to the personality of the male or female subjects. However, total cholesterol was 200 mg/dl for males who repress and deny experiencing anxiety and emotions, compared to 160 mg/dl for males who are honest with themselves and others and who are less defensive about reporting that they experience anxiety. For females, cholesterol was unrelated to personality. Although it is not understood why personality influenced the cholesterol level for the men and not the women, anxiety or anger may play an important and deadly role in triggering the transport of fat out of storage and into the bloodstream while people are under stress. Perhaps individuals who repress their emotions mobilize more fat and have a more exaggerated physiological response to stressful situations than others do. This could drive up cholesterol levels and create more opportunities over time for the buildup of plaque in the arteries.

In a related study, Shari Waldstein and associates at the University of Pittsburgh examined the relationship of several dimensions of anger and its expression to fasting total cholesterol and lipoprotein concentrations.[88] The subjects for this study were 29 healthy white males (average age, 24) who also completed the Spielbeger Trait Anger and Anger Expression Scales; the latter instrument subsumes three subscales termed: anger-out; anger-in; and anger-control.

The results of this study revealed a significant positive correlation between anger-out and HDL ($r = .46$). In addition, trait anger correlated significantly with HDL ($r = .34$) while anger-control was inversely related to HDL ($r = -.37$). These results demonstrate a moderate relationship between fasting HDL cholesterol concentrations and both the experience (trait anger) and outward (anger-out) expression of anger. On the other hand, a reluctance to acknowledge or express anger (anger-control) is associated with a relatively lower (i.e., potentially deleterious) HDL concentration.

Psychologist Edward Suarez and his colleagues at Duke University Medical Center have discovered that Type-A men with elevated cholesterol show an exaggerated reactivity to stress that could lead to heart attacks[89]. In this study, changes in levels of adrenaline, noradrenaline, and cortisol—chemicals that rise when people are emotionally upset and experiencing stress—were measured both in healthy, hard-driving Type-A men of middle age and their easy-going Type-B counterparts. As the results of this study indicate, in Type-As with high cholesterols (200–300 mg/dl), the chemicals reflective of stress rose above their usual levels when the men were performing a mentally stressful task. On the other hand, two of the stress chemicals fell below their usual levels in the easygoing Type B men. Overall, these findings suggest that, in persons who are already at risk for cardiovascular disease because of high cholesterol levels, personality may determine those persons whose arteries are under greater stress and may be more sensitive to damage to the inner lining.

Such findings are particularly interesting in view of the significant relationship between hostility and LDL cholesterol values in men and women that has been reported by Ulf Lundberg and associates.[87] The participants in this case were nonsmoking healthy white-collar workers (middle managers and clerical workers) in Sweden. Most importantly, the results showed that only hostility scores were significantly associated with excessive physiological reactivity to stress and with LDL cholesterol values in both men and women.

To summarize, the relationship between the AHA! Syndrome and both hypertension and coronary heart disease seems a bit topsy-turvy. On the one hand, suppressed anger (Anger-In) and submissiveness are related to elevated blood pressure and hypertension in many studies. Given the cross-sectional nature of most studies, however, it is difficult to argue specifically for the predictive role of suppressed anger.[79] In other words, it is difficult to determine whether suppressed anger (or any other components of the AHA! Syndrome) precedes or is a consequence of hypertension. On the other hand, it seems that high levels of hostility and outwardly expressed anger (Anger-Out) contribute to heart disease in general, and to coronary heart disease in particular. So what is it that we can safely conclude? The truth is that the experience and expression (or lack of expression) of anger and hostility in extreme forms are associated with an increased risk for cardiovascular disease as well as with certain classic risk factors for heart disease. What the exact relative risk is, and the consistency of the relationship between the AHA! Syndrome and the classic risk factors are matters that may soon be revealed by the studies currently in progress.

4

Cancers, Ulcers, Smoking, and Psoriasis

This chapter reviews the research literature relating stress and emotional factors to cancer, ulcers, smoking, and psoriasis. Although psychosocial stress and emotional factors have been reported to play a role in their onset or maintenance, the available research connecting elements of the AHA! Syndrome to these conditions is not so great as that for hypertension and cardiovascular diseases. Therefore, all four conditions will be examined in a single chapter.

PSYCHOSOCIAL FACTORS AND CANCER

It has been suggested that the onset of cancer occurs more in some personality types than others and that certain personality factors are associated with a poorer prognosis once cancer has been diagnosed. Unlike the studies showing links between hypertension (and CHD) and elements of the AHA! Syndrome, research linking psychosocial or personality factors to cancer has not gained much acceptance. Nevertheless, a number of clinical studies relating certain patterns of dealing with stress and personality type with the development of cancer have been published over the past 25 years. One of the pioneers, Lawrence LeShan studied more than 400 cancer patients during the 1960s. After spending an enormous amount of time in psychotherapy with each of 71 patients, he found that approximately 72 percent had lost an important relationship before their cancers appeared. Further studies by LeShan revealed that the typical cancer patient experiences difficulty in forming close relationships and generally has lost either a parent or a sibling early in childhood. For unknown reasons, the cancer patients blame themselves and feel quite abandoned and lonely over the loss of these close primary relationships; and they tend to repress these feelings and deny their importance.

In another study, Caroline Thomas of Johns Hopkins University studied more than 1,000 students annually to determine whether emotional and psychological factors would contribute to diseases 14 years later in life.[2,3] To her surprise, she found that cancer patients were submissive and not aggressive, and experience many difficulties in their relationships with family members—particularly their fathers—early in their lives. Moreover, the psychological profiles of the individuals who developed cancer were quite similar to the students who became mentally ill or committed suicide. Subsequent reports of these data using additional methods to measure "closeness to parents" have revealed that the degree to which early relationships are "unbalanced" is a predictor of cancer even after considering smoking, serum cholesterol level, and age at the onset of the study.[3-5] Other studies conducted over the years have confirmed these observations. For example, William Green's studies of patients with leukemia and lymphoma led him to conclude that, in nine cases out of ten, the development of the cancer occurred within individuals who felt depressed, helpless, hopeless, and alone— generally soon after they experienced the loss of an important primary and close relationship.[7] In another study David Kissen of the University of Glasgow found that the risk of lung cancer was five times higher among male heavy smokers who had poor and inadequate outlets for emotional expression than among heavy smokers with good emotional outlets and strong bonds with family members and close friends.[7]

One prospective study first reported in 1975[8] by researchers S. Green and associates at the Faith Courtland Unit for Studies in Cancer at Kings College Hospital in London later indicated that the psychological responses exhibited by women following the diagnosis of breast cancer were related to length of survival five[9] and ten[10] years later. Briefly, the women who reacted to cancer by denial or a fighting spirit had a more favorable outcome than those patients who responded with a stoic acceptance or feelings of helplessness or hopelessness. Subsequent findings at the 10-year follow-up showed that psychological response was independent of all other prognostic variables and was the most significant individual factor in determining both recurrence of breast cancer and death. Green and his associates also found that women who either suppressed their feelings of anger or who turned it inward against themselves and became depressed were more likely to have malignant breast lumps than women who were able to express their anger. Interestingly, women who habitually and chronically suppressed their feelings of anger had higher blood levels of an antibody that was elevated in patients with cancer.[11]

As recently as 1988, the team of researchers at the Faith Courtland Unit published findings based on 168 newly diagnosed patients in order to replicate their earlier research with breast cancer.[12,13] In their current study, they attempted to extend the investigation to a type of malignancy—Hodgkin's lymphoma—that would include men. With regard to breast cancer among women, the recent study confirmed their previous findings that psychological response to cancer is independent of other known prognostic factors. In particular, there was no evidence of any association between psychological response and local lymph-node involvement.

In both Hodgkin's and non-Hodgkin's lymphoma patients, there was evidence of greater psychiatric morbidity—as reflected by their levels of anxiety and depression—among those patients with a more advanced form of the cancer and those who failed to respond to treatment. However, no association was found between any psychological response and any clinical or pathological variable. Moreover, there was no evidence that the patient's gender or type of tumor affected her or his overall psychological adjustment to cancer, or that the effect noted among breast cancer patients might possibly apply to all types of malignant disease. A determination of the relationship between psychological responses and the survival of patients must await future inquiry, since these patients were examined only 3–12 months following the diagnosis of cancer.

In another study conducted in the early 1980s, Lydia Temoshok—a psychologist at the University of California at San Francisco—performed psychological assessments of 150 middle-aged melanoma patients to study the link between cancer and personality traits.[14] Her findings showed that a large number of these patients did not express negative emotions. Even in the face of cancer, they maintained an even temperament—almost never venting their anger, sadness, depression, or fear. One of the most important findings obtained from this study was that those patients who expressed emotions more openly were often found to have less aggressive tumor growth and stronger immunologic responses and were less likely to relapse than patients who had difficulties expressing their emotions. There is also a hint here that the psychological factors played a role chiefly among younger patients, while age-related factors seem more important for predicting outcome following cancer diagnosis among older patients.

Temoshok recently compared the coping styles of cancer patients (those with malignant melanoma), patients with cardiovascular disease, and healthy controls.[15] In this study, subjects were characterized as having a "repressive coping style" if, during exposure to an anger- and anxiety-provoking situation, they did not become upset but their physiological response was elevated. In this context, patients with malignant melanomas demonstrated a greater degree of repressive coping than the other groups.

Other recent studies of women with and without breast cancer have found that natural killer (NK) cell activity is lower—which decreases the capacity of controlling the spread of micrometastases—among breast cancer patients who are rated as being not well adjusted.[16,17] Similarly, NK activity is lower among those women who have a less than desirable degree of support in their environment, and those who are characterized as being listless, apathetic, and lacking in vigor. NK cell activity has also been related to psychological health in a study made of healthy college students by J.S. Heisel and colleagues.[16] In this study, students who had high levels of NK activity had a psychologically healthier profile on scales of the MMPI than did students with low NK activity levels. In another recent study of patients with malignant melanoma, S.M. Levy found a positive relationship between survival and both active NK cells and high scores on a questionnaire that assessed mood profile, and a negative relationship between survival and the belief called "negative attribution"—that whatever happens will be for the worst.[17] Although the sample was small (13 patients), these factors—NK activity, positive mood, and absence of belief in negative attribution—predicted survival in nearly half of the patients.

Recent evidence of the connection between psychological factors and mortality from cancer can also be seen in two studies conducted in Europe and the Uniter States. The first study was reported in 1985 by Ronald Grossarth-Maticek, Jan Bastiaans, and Dusan Kanazir.[18] This team of researchers investigated the relation of psychosocial risk factors to mortality in a prospective study among 1,353 inhabitants of Crvenka, Yugoslavia—619 of whom died between 1966 and 1976. Overall, the 38 individuals who died from lung cancer, and 29 whose deaths were due to other cancers, were characterized by having high scores on "rationality" and "antiemotionality"—psychological measures that connoted suppression of aggression and hostility. Most interestingly, when all of the data were adjusted for the degree of rationality and antiemotionality, the relationship between smoking and lung cancer was reduced, and the relationship between smoking and other forms of cancer as well as the relationship between smoking and heart disease was virtually eliminated. Furthermore, the Yugoslav researchers discovered that feelings of long-lasting hopelessness and depression at the beginning of the study were independently associated with incidence of cancer, as was anger with heart disease. Although these results are regarded by some as being too good to be true, other researchers—most notably Hans J. Eysenck—do view Grossarth-Maticek's research as being scientifically valid.[19] A similar study started in 1972 in Heidelberg Germany, followed 1,273 "stressed" subjects and 872 "normal" subjects more than ten years.[20] Whereas this work largely replicated the findings of the Yugoslav study, the Heidelberg findings have also been criticized—mostly because of the way its subjects were selected.

The second study involved a 20-year follow-up of 2,018 employees of the Western Electric Company and was reported in 1987 by Victoria Persky, Joan Kempthorne-Rawson, and Richard Shekelle.[21] In this study, psychologic depression as measured by the MMPI was found to be positively associated with 20-year incidence and mortality from cancer. The association was not stronger for one type of cancer than another, but it did appear to be stronger for the risk of fatal cancer than for total cancer incidence. Furthermore, the association between psychologic depression and the incidence of cancer was apparent only during the first ten years of the follow-up, while the association with mortality was observed for the full 20 years of the follow-up. These results are consistent with previous studies showing that depression may promote the development and spread of malignant neoplasms. For example, in 1954 E.M. Blumberg found that patients with rapidly progressing tumors were more likely to have high levels of depression, compared with patients with less aggressive tumors.[22] Dr. Blumberg also noted that patients with fast-growing tumors were the most eager to present their best face to the world at all times and have people think well of them. In other words, they exhibited denial.

Although there have been many great strides in the legitimacy of psychosomatic medicine and medical psychology in the past decade, most physicians still only pay lip service to the idea that negative emotions can have anything more than a transient effect on the muscles, tissues, and organs that make up the human body. Besides, level of emotional discomfort is far less observable and quantifiable than the size of a tumor, and the pathways between the two remain unclear. Furthermore, when you consider the solidity of nerves, muscles, and flesh beneath the thin covering of skin, you wonder (as I did when I had surgery to remove a nonmalignant growth) how emotions and thoughts— intangible and unmeasurable—can alter the biochemistry and physical structure of the body to the point of developing cancerous tumors. Yet there are hundreds of articles in the medical and psychological literature discussing the linkages between personality, emotions, and stress and the development of neoplasia.

Personally, I think that the greatest advancements in this area are coming from studies that examine the mechanisms connecting psychological processes and immunity and disease susceptibility. For example, the recent reviews of the role of depressed immune function in the development of cancer clearly indicate that psychological factors— particularly depression (which could, as discussed in Chapter 3, be anger turned inward)—may increase promotion of cancer by altering the immune system and decreasing the ability to reject malignant cells.[23,24] Some of the most impressive research to date is being conducted at the Ohio State University College of Medicine.[25,26] These studies are directed under the leadership of psychologist Janice Kiecolt-Glaser and her husband, immunologist Ronald Glaser. Basically, the Glasers and their research team have focused their attention on the relationship between marital disruption and immune function.

The rationale for this focus has to do with the fact that marital quality is the single most powerful sociodemographic predictor of stress-related physical illness, with separated persons having approximately 30 percent more acute illness and physician visits than married people. Men and women who are separated or divorced have poorer mental and physical health than their counterparts who are remarried or who were widowed, or those who remain single. Furthermore, separated and divorced individuals have the highest rates of chronic medical conditions that are associated with disability and a limiting of social activities. Recent studies also show that bereavement is associated with poor immune functioning. For example, bereaved spouses have a poorer lymphocyte proliferative response to mitogen stimulation several weeks after their spouse's death than nonbereaved subjects, and men whose wives were dying of breast cancer showed poorer lymphocyte proliferation after their spouse's death than prior to the death.[24]

In a report published in January 1987, the Glasers compared the psychologic and immune function measures of 38 married women and 38 separated/divorced women. Among married women, poorer marital quality was related to greater psychologic depression and poorer immune function (e.g., a lower percentage of NK cells and helper T cells). Women who had been separated one year or less had significantly poorer immune function than their married counterparts. Moreover, the separated/divorced women who were separated for the shortest period of time and who had a greater preoccupation with and negative attachment to their ex-husband had poorer immune function and a greater level of psychologic depression.

In another study published as in May 1988, the Glasers compared psychologic and immune function measures of 32 married men and 32 separated/divorced men.[26] The results of their comparison showed that separated and divorced men were more distressed and lonelier, and reported significantly more recent illnesses than married men. Separated and divorced men also had significantly poorer values on several indexes of immunity. Among married men, poorer marital quality was associated with greater psychological distress, a poorer response on functional immunologic measures, and lower helper/suppressor T cell ratios. Taken together, the pattern of these findings indicate that the quality of one's interpersonal relationships do have health-related consequences. The Glasers concluded that an increase in psychological distress as from a chronically abrasive marital relationship can lead to adverse immunological changes. Furthermore, these immunological changes may explain why psychologic distress related to the loss of important relationships leads to an increased incidence of infectious disease.

Given this framework, then, how one copes with and expresses intense feelings of irritability and anger within problematic interpersonal relationships may be directly related to immune system irregularities, with the end result being a reduced ability to reject tumors. In other words, women and men who express their anger might experience less disruptions in the functioning of their immune system than those who suppress strong feelings of anger. Unfortunately, information about anger–hostility coping styles was not collected in the studies by the Glasers. Future research should be directed to this issue.

As noted briefly in Chapter 2, one of the pathways between the growth of tumors and the emotional reaction to stress involves activation of the limbic system, which stimulates the hypothalamus—that part of the brain most directly associated with emotions. In this sequence of events, the hypothalamus activates the pituitary to stimulate the adrenal cortex, which floods the body with adrenal hormones (epinephrine, norepinephrine, etc.). These hormones help to prepare the body for action and to deal with the negative emotional reaction to stress—the fight-or-flight response. Unfortunately, action is not often possible for many of us in these modern times. It is seldom advisable to express anger openly and blow-up at a boss or a co-worker. And no matter how loud we scream during a traffic jam, it will not make heavy traffic move faster. The end result of our practical inhibitions, however, is that the adrenal hormones circulate in our bodies at a higher concentration for a longer period of time, affecting the immune system in at least two ways: (1) There occurs a decrease in the number of T cells due to shrinkage of the thymus—the origin of the T cells; and (2) The imbalance in the adrenal hormones creates an overall depression of the immune system and a corresponding increase in the body's production of abnormal cells and in susceptibility to carcinogens.

Although the etiology of chronic anger and hostility is largely unknown, interpersonal conflict centered around divorce—particularly a contested divorce—appears to be one area that serves as a catalyst for heated arguments and fights between men and women. Moreover, as revealed by the work of the Glasers, going through a divorce is such a powerful and stressful event that it disrupts the functioning of the immune system for some women and men.

Whereas the Glasers did not measure how women express and suppress feelings of anger and hostility, their 1987 research did clearly show the that women with the strongest attachment to their ex-husbands had the poorest immune function. Could it be that attachment to the ex-husbands resulted in anger, resentment, and hostile attitudes that were prolonged or regenerated by recalling and focusing on the stressfulness of the divorce? The answer is probably yes, and it is highly probable that these situations disturb the body's immune mechanisms in proportion to the intensity and duration of the memory of the negative emotional states. Also, whether anger and other elements of the AHA! Syndrome are acknowledged and expressed, or repressed, is critical in the development of disease. For example—as indicated in this chapter— among women with breast cancer, the ability to communicate feelings of anger and talk openly about their psychological distress is related to the length of survival after the diagnosis of cancer. Although the findings presented above support theories of interaction between immune status and mental stress, the mechanisms and direction of interaction remain largely unexplored.

THE SIMONTON APPROACH

Another approach to studying the link between emotions and cancer has emerged from the psychological treatment of cancer that was developed by O. Carl Simonton and Stephanie Mathews-Simonton.[27] This treatment program combines orthodox medical therapy with meditation, visualization, and both individual and group psychotherapy. The visualization technique is an ancient one similar to those used in meditational disciplines. Basically, the cancer patients are taught how to relax their entire body, and then to visualize themselves in a very pleasant and peaceful environment. Once relaxed the patients are then instructed to picture their cancer cells as disorganized, weak, and more vulnerable than normal cells, and to picture the white cells destroying and carrying off the dead cancer cells. Patients are also directed to picture whatever conventional treatment they are receiving (e.g., radiation therapy) as attacking and destroying the cancer cells without harming healthy cells. In other cases, the visualization involves patients' seeing their own immune systems as being strong and aggressively fighting and destroying the cancer cells which are flushed away.

Although the Simontons point out that visualization has a number of benefits—helping patients to focus on healing; reducing anxiety; increasing the awareness of the unity of mind and body; lowering the physiological state of arousal—this is only one part of the total program. There are at least six aspects of the Simonton program that include visualization and meditation techniques, group and individual psychotherapy, exercise, and a continuation of whatever orthodox medical therapy the patient has been receiving. The first thing the Simontons do, however, is to weed out all but the cancer patients who are most determined to succeed and benefit from the program. In other words, there is a concerted effort to enroll only those patients with a positive attitude toward treatment and who have goals for living, a will to live, and a strong and positive belief that they will live through their cancer.

The patients are also required to bring their spouse or closest family member or best friend, so that on returning home the patient will have the needed support and understanding of someone who knows the program. During the 10-day stay at a special clinic, participants are involved in an intensive program including daily meditations and visualizations. Patients are encouraged to set short- and long-term goals based on the assumption that they will recover from the cancer. In the group and individual psychotherapy sessions that are also part of the daily program, patients are taught how to combat negative emotional states and how to cope with the fears that many cancer patients experience—fears of recurrence, disability, and death. Patients are also taught how to manage feelings of anger and hostility, and how to express them openly and effectively. Finally, the Simontons require their patients to engage in a regular physical exercise and fitness program—the rationale here being that people who engage regularly in exercise programs tend to be less depressed, anxious, and worried.

Since the start-up of their program in the early 1970s the Simontons have trained more than 5,000 health professionals in the utilization of their treatment techniques. For the most part, the statistics compiled by the Simontons in their book Getting Well Again are nothing less than impressive. For example, among 240 "incurable" cancer patients who were treated by the Simontons between 1973 and 1979, the median survival time has been double that of the average for the nation. Also, about 10 percent of the patients they treated had a dramatic remission of their cancers.   Nevertheless, the findings have been criticized by many researchers, and the American Cancer Society has found no evidence that the Simonton program provides objective benefit other than that it promotes relaxation, a sense of control, and psychological well-being.

Work similar to the Simontons has been conducted by a number of other individuals. For example, B. Siegel presented no data but reported many anecdotes about patients in whom deliberately evoked feelings of self-love and love of others were soon followed by at least a temporary— and sometimes permanent—regression of apparently terminal cancers.[28] In the early 1980s, B.W. Newton described a program much like the Simontons, but with an emphasis on hypnosis.[29] Depending on the site of the cancers, patients had median survival lengths 2.5–4 times that of the national medians. Ronald Grossarth-Maticek also exposed cancer patients to what he referred to as "social psychotherapy" and promoted a healthy lifestyle, natural piety, expression of goals and hopes, and trust in and support from the physician and other people important to the patient.[30] Results of this investigation revealed that patients exposed to this form of therapy had median survival times two years longer than controls matched for cancer type, age, sex, and social class.

In summary, there appears to be good evidence in support of the involvement of psychosocial factors in the development of cancer. Although important stressful life circumstances are always associated with cancer, it seems that how a person copes with and handles stress is more important than the source of the stress. Several studies have identified a constellation of emotional, cognitive, and behavioral traits—including suppressed anger–hostility and unbalanced interpersonal relationships—believed to alter severely the biological homeostasis and to increase the susceptibility to development of cancer. However, the biologic and physiologic pathways whereby these unpleasant circumstances contribute to disease is still a bit unclear.

PSYCHOLOGICAL CHARACTERISTICS OF ULCER PATIENTS

The importance of psychological factors in the pathogenesis of peptic ulcers was once widely accepted.[31–34] Over the years, there have been many confirmations that emotional stresses, fatigue, and mental worry and anxiety coincided with the presence of gastric ulceration. For example, in 1929 and 1930 W.C. Alvaraz noted that certain types of people are more prone to develop peptic ulcers (resulting from the action of digestive juices) than other people.[32] During this same era, Howard Hartman characterized the individual with ulcers as a man who is "encountering obstacles that prove him a trial and handicap, which he must, because of his nature, endeavor to overcome."[33] The peptic ulcers had long been considered a disease of the civilized world because it afflicted men living in the Western culture, which encourages them to be ambitious and striving chronically to achieve more and more out of their available time. Hartman went a bit further to claim that certain groups of people (e.g., the Chinese and Latin American Indians) may never develop ulcers because of their "stoic and almost apathetic attitude" and the lack of strain that characterize these groups.

Various authors have reported a significant relationship between the onset of symptoms of peptic ulcers and domestic problems, financial and economic hardships, or a long past history of anxiety and stress. In 1957, F. Avery Jones found that anxiety, frustration, resentment, and fatigue are aggravating factors in the symptomatology of peptic ulceration.[34] At the time, much of what was known about the linkages between emotional factors and gastrointestinal disturbances such as ulcers was derived from studies conducted by Franz Alexander and his colleagues at the Chicago Institute for Psychoanalysis.[35] These studies clearly revealed that gastric symptoms, including peptic ulcers, develop more frequently in one personality type than in others. However, there were many exceptions—which led this impressive group of clinical researchers to derive the following conclusion.

> In overt behavior many peptic-ulcer patients show an exaggerated aggressive, ambitious, independent attitude. They do not like to accept help and burden themselves with all kinds of responsibilities—the type that is so often seen among efficient business executives. The continuous struggle and excessive responsibilities reinforce the wish for a dependent relationship. He carefully hides this dependent attitude from himself, however, and represses it so that it cannot find expression in overt behavior. This repressed longing for love is the unconscious psychological stimulus directly connected with the physiological processes leading finally to ulceration. It would appear that the crucial factor in the pathogenesis of ulcer is the frustration of the dependent, help-seeking, and love-demanding desires. When these desires cannot find

gratification in human relationships, a chronic emotional stimulus is created which has a specific effect upon the functions of the stomach. (Alexander 1987, pp. 102–3)[35]

It is not certain that the catalyst for the typical conflict situation described by Alexander and his colleagues is always a frustration of dependent desires. There is, however, much evidence in support of the notion that one causative factor in ulcer formation may be the frequent and continuous hypersecretion of gastric juices and acids during psychologically and emotionally stressful periods. Moreover, it has been suggested that these chronic emotional and psychological disturbances to the empty stomach are similar to what naturally occurs during the digestion of food. Alexander and his colleagues supported their theory with several case histories of ulcer patients, rather than controlled experiments. Given the quantity and yet lack of quality of many studies published these days, one wonders whether the problems associated with clinical case studies are worse than the problems we face today.

One of the first studies to investigate experimentally the influence of emotions on gastric activity was conducted by Bela Mittelmann and Harold Wolff in 1942.[36] They induced acute emotional disturbances in ulcer patients and in normal patients without ulcers. During this induction, the ulcer patients exhibited a larger increase in hydrochloric acid, mucus, and pepsin secretions than the patients without ulcers. Patients with ulcers also experienced more pain, increased bile secretion, and bleeding in response to the experimentally induced frustration—which was designed to elicit feelings of anxiety, irritability and guilt. Mittelmann and Wolff went a bit further and subjected these same patients to situations that were not stressful or frustrating, and where there was a greater degree of emotional security. In these situations, gastric functions were found to be normal and not significantly different from the patients without ulcers.

In 1957 Herbert Weiner and his colleagues (Margaret Thaler, Morton Reiser, and Arthur Mirsky) published one of the most well conceived studies ever to examine the relationship between specific psychological characteristics and the rate of gastric secretion—in this case, serum pepsinogen.[37] Over the years, many studies had shown that the concentration of pepsinogen in the bloodstream is dependent on the rate of pepsinogen production in the stomach and that, in approximately 90 percent of patients with duodenal ulcers, pepsinogen concentrations are substantially greater than in patients without duodenal ulcers or gastrointestinal disturbances. Moreover, the concentration of pepsinogen and the increased rate of gastric secretion continues to be high in ulcer patients after the ulcer is healed. This fact led Dr. Weiner and his group to conclude that the gastric hypersecretion is essential but not the sole determinant of the development of the ulcer, and that perhaps psychological factors and the regular occurrence of psychosocial stress contribute to the onset of ulcers.

The Weiner study team randomly selected a group of 63 men with the highest level of gastric secretion and compared them with a group of 57 men who had the lowest pepsinogen values. The men were selected from among 2,073 draftees (age 18–29 years) who were being processed at an army camp in the northeastern United States. During the 16-week basic training, the men in both of these study groups underwent a series of medical and psychological examinations. The major finding was that all subjects who had or developed evidence of a duodenal ulcer were in the group of men with the highest blood pepsinogen values. Without any knowledge of the pepsinogen values, one psychologist and two psychiatrists independently rated the psychological test data to determine whether each subject had a high or low blood concentration of pepsinogen. On the basis of a majority opinion, 85 percent of the men could be correctly classified. And the psychological data revealed that subjects with peptic ulcers displayed evidence of major unresolved and persistent conflicts about dependency and oral gratification. Whereas ulcer patients do try to satisfy these needs in various ways, when such attempts fail they experience a high level of frustration that will arouse strong feelings of anger—feelings that are not openly expressed because of the potential loss of sources for gratifying their dependency needs. Consequently, the ulcer patient becomes submissive and passive, does not make complaints, and is prone to hostile impulses that are felt but not revealed or directly expressed.

In a report in 1970, M.H. Alp, J.H. Court, and A.K. Grant completed a retrospective survey of 181 patients who had been admitted with chronic gastric ulceration to two major public hospitals in South Australia between 1954 and 1963.[38] In this group of 181 participants there was a significantly increased incidence of domestic and financial stress when compared to a group of 181 persons who had no history of gastric ulcer. The researchers found that individuals with chronic gastric ulcer are characterized by a personality pattern of independence and self-sufficiency, and that they are prone to experience intense feelings of anxiety and depression and to behave in a submissive manner—probably because they fear and avoid the clashes or social disapproval that would result from assertive-hostile behavior toward others.

While the significance of emotional factors in the etiology of peptic ulcer is widely accepted by the public, there is divergence of opinion concerning how this process works. In a very important investigation, Arthur Mirsky and his colleagues designed a study that would permit the measurement of gastric activity and accompanying emotional stress associated with the usual day-to-day events in men over long periods of time.[37,39] It had been demonstrated previously that the rate of gastric secretion can be determined by the amount of pepsinogen in the urine. In this study, a simultaneous record of daily events was maintained, along with daily urine analysis to determine the level of pepsinogen. Mirsky concluded that overt anger, frustration, resentment, and a variety of other dominant emotions reported by the subjects did not significantly influence the degree of gastric activity.[39] However, a positive relationship was observed between an increase in gastric activity as reflected by excretion of pepsinogen, and subjects' fear of losing a significant dependent relationship.

In a study published in 1982, G. Lykestos and colleagues compared the personality traits and the states of anxiety and depression in a group of duodenal ulcer patients and a group of hypertensive patients against a control group of other physically ill patients at admission and discharge.[40] Both the ulcer and the hypertensive patients were more submissive and more anxious than the control group at admission to the medical center, while the ulcer patients were less depressed and anxious than the hypertensive patients. At discharge, both the ulcer and the hypertensive patients continued to be more submissive and more anxious than the group of patients in the control group, and the ulcer patients remained less submissive and less anxious than the hypertensives. With improvement in their physical symptoms during their stay at the medical center, both the ulcer and the hypertensive patients became less depressed, but there was no change in their anxiety levels. Basically, the overall pattern of other findings shows that the ulcer and the hypertensive patients reported more dependent behavior as lifelong characteristics when compared to the control group, and the results support the hypothesis that personality conflicts relating to competitive hostility and dependence play a role in psychosomatic disease.

From the standpoint of the "psychodynamic theory of repressed hostility," peptic ulcers are believed to be the result of the following complex chain of events: 1) frustration of oral-receptive longing > (2) oral-aggressive responses > (3) guilt > (4) anxiety > (5) overcompensation for oral aggression and dependence by successful accomplishments in responsible activities > (6) increased unconscious oral-dependent cravings as reaction to excessive effort and concentration > (7) gastric hypersecretion.[41]

On the other hand, hypertension is thought to result from a different chain of events: (1) hostile competitive traits > (2) intimidation due to fear of retaliation > (3) increase of dependent longings > (4) inferiority feelings > (5) reactivation of hostile competitiveness > (6) anxiety and resultant inhibition of aggressive hostile impulses > (7) hypertension.[41,42]

These sequences of events remind me of the scene in the movie The Verdict where Paul Newman, portraying a not too happy or sober lawyer, is offered $210,000 as the out-of-court settlement for a case involving medical malpractice. In the movie, there is no doubt that Newman needs the money; but his response to the lawyers representing the hospital is something like, "It's interesting how this figure is so neatly divided by three." In the end, he refuses to settle out of court and goes on to win the case. I think it's interesting how there are seven components in the psychodynamic chain of events leading to the onset or development of both ulcers and hypertension—as if there were some kind of biblical undertone, maybe, to this notion of seven stages. Don't get me wrong: I am not saying that there is anything wrong with the scheme or that this psychodynamic view should be abandoned. Quite simply, however, the two dynamic patterns have common denominators that could be rephrased in other terms. For example, angry–hostile– aggressive tendencies of the AHA! Syndrome can be perceived as causing personal conflicts such that feelings of anxiety and guilt associated with the recognition of these tendencies—presumably viewed as unacceptable traits—increase the presence of submissiveness and feelings of anger and other hostile emotions, which become suppressed rather than result in increased aggressiveness, dominance, or the free-and-easy outward expression of anger. In other words, the patients with ulcers and hypertension behave like neurotics.

Be that as it may, clinical research on personality factors related to the onset, maintenance, and worsening of ulcers is plentiful. Critical reviews of the psychosocial "causes" of ulcers continue to be published. This field of psychosomatic research—much like studies of hypertension and cancer—suffers because of the notably diverse number of psychological instruments used to measure various personality disturbances. Although there are a number of other problems that make it difficult to determine the role of personality factors in ulcers, the analyses of the studies published show that there is nevertheless a certain level of agreement. For example, a review of 76 articles on psychosomatic factors and peptic ulcer disease by G. Magni and colleagues revealed that: (1) peptic ulcer patients are often characterized by a personality with dependence/independence problems and high levels of anxiety and irritability; (2) data concerning the role of stress appear to be far from uniform and often even contradictory; and (3) although much remains to be done with respect to the possible link between psychological and biological parameters, the results concerning the relationship between psyche and secretory patterns are very interesting and represent one of the most important lines of future research.[42]

This review prompted Magni to formulate and conduct one of the most interesting studies in this area of research. Forty patients with duodenal ulcers were monitored to determine whether personality and psychological factors are associated with biological parameters related to slow-healing and reoccurrence of ulcer. Results indicated that the patients with elevated maximal stomach-acid output and elevated total serum pepsinogen values showed an anxiety and irritability level that was significantly greater than patients with low gastric-acid concentration.

In another recent study by Magni and the group of Italian researchers, the relationship between personality and duodenal ulcer response to antisecretory treatment was examined to determine whether psychological factors are related to relapse.[42] One group of patients—the responders—were characterized by not having a proven relapse during treatment with antisecretory drugs for a period of 12 months after healing of the lesion. Nonresponders were all patients with at least one relapse during treatment with antisecretory drugs. Analysis of psychological data as measured by the Cattell 16 Personality Factor Questionnaire,[43] indicated that the group of duodenal ulcer patients with personality marked by high levels of dominance, dependence, neuroticism, and anxiety traits were more prone to relapse. The significance of this Magni study becomes even more clear in light of the 1988 review of psychosocial causes of duodenal ulcer, by C. Tennant.[44] According to this review, a variety of both experimental stressors and different emotional states (such as anxiety, irritability, and anger) are related to increased gastric acid and pepsin secretion. Furthermore, patients with high levels of anxiety or neuroticism are more prone to stress-induced anxiety and its physiological consequence—which often include an increased gastric-acid output. Given that approximately 40 percent of duodenal ulcer patients relapse in the first year after medical treatment, there seems to be a strong place here for psychological treatments, especially in the domain of managing exaggerated emotional responses to stress. This appears to be especially true for those patients who relapse or those patients characterized by high levels of anxiety, neuroticism, and dependence.

The psychological characteristics of patients with gastric and duodenal ulcer disease have been assessed in several recent studies. Basically, the findings show that patients with gastric ulcers have higher neuroticism, hostility, and depression scores than patients with duodenal ulcers. The psychological profiles of the two ulcer groups in relation to healthy individuals without ulcers show that duodenal ulcer patients have higher introversion and psychoticism scores, while gastric ulcer patients have higher anxiety and psychoticism scores. Therefore, these findings can be taken to indicate that there are subtle differences in the emotional states of patients with different ulcers, but they are similar with regard to deeper or underlying personality conflicts. For example, Mark Feldman and colleagues demonstrated that ulcer patients and controls experience a similar number of potentially stressful life events.[45,46] However, ulcer patients perceive their events more negatively and have more personality disturbances and emotional distress as reflected by increased depression and anxiety. Ulcer patients are also pessimistic, and excessively dependent, and they have fewer friends and relatives whom they feel they can call on for help in times of crisis.

In most of the studies that I have examined, the ulcer patients tend to be hypochondriacally complainers, overly pessimistic, excessively dependent, immature, and impulsive, and have a significantly lower ego strength. Similarly, comparisons of the psychological profiles of peptic ulcer patients and those with other gastrointestinal disorders such as irritable bowel syndrome have shown that the personality profiles are essentially the same, but that patients from both groups differ from normal populations.[42] From a psychosomatic point of view, patients with irritable bowel syndrome and peptic ulcers may be viewed as presenting different biological facets of the same underlying psychological conflicts. In any case, it does seem reasonable to consider psychological and emotional stress reactions of patients with gastrointestinal disorders when formulating treatment programs.

One of the major problems with examining the relationship between personality factors and ulcers is that the psychological data—high levels of anxiety, neuroticism, anger, and so forth—may be as much reactions to the gastrointestinal disorder as they are causal agents. To counteract this problem, several studies of duodenal ulcer patients have been conducted to differentiate subgroups based on age at disease onset.[42] In most of these studies, a group of patients suffering from chronic recurrent duodenal ulcers is subdivided into two groups according to whether the first manifestations of the disorder occurred early or late in the life of each patient. Comparisons of the two groups often reveal that the patients in Group I (early manifestation) have a larger number of constitutional handicaps along with a higher incidence of dispositional experience with regard to loss of significant family members, and they assumed social responsibility at an early age. Patients in Group II (late manifestation) are often characterized by a larger number of depressive symptoms, a higher incidence of alcohol abuse, and attempts at suicide. Overall, patients in Group I frequently exhibit the characteristics of the ulcer type described by Franz Alexander (i.e., stemming from frustrated dependency),[35] as well as chronic anger; while patients from Group II suffer from depressed disorders that have affected their personalities.

A 1988 study reported by Pamela Walker and colleagues is interesting in this regard.[46] In their study, Pamela Walker and her colleagues examined whether psychological disturbances in men with peptic ulcer disease might be related to other potential ulcer risk factors: serum pepsinogen concentrations, cigarette smoking, and intake of alcohol, coffee, or aspirin. In a general sense, increased emotional disturbances, hostility, irritability, hypersensitivity, and impaired coping ability (i.e., a negative perception of life events) each correlated significantly with increased serum pepsinogen concentration in ulcer patients. Although cigarette smoking, and the intake of alcohol and aspirin were increased in ulcer patients, they were unrelated to increased emotional disturbances or psychopathology. Overall, depression was the variable that best discriminated ulcer patients from nonulcer control subjects; and the findings support the notion that emotional stress may predispose to ulcers by producing gastric hypersecretion, as manifested by hyperpepsinogenemia.

In summary, the studies on the psychological characteristics of ulcer patients do not clearly show that personality and psychological factors cause either ulcers or the increased level of gastric acid secretions that often accompany ulcers. However, the consistency of the associations between certain personality/psychological factors and both the output of gastric acids and ulcers makes it difficult to argue against the involvement of psychic factors in ulcers. There appears to be strong support for the notion that chronic ulcer patients struggle with issues regarding dependence and exaggerated aggressiveness, and that psychological factors such as anxiety and neuroticism relate to elevated stomach acid levels reflective of the rate of gastric secretion. Interesting research regarding the relationship between personality and relapse among ulcer patients receiving medical (pharmacologic) treatment has revealed that ulcer patients with personality characterized by high levels of anxiety and irritability, dependence problems, and neuroticism are more prone to relapse. This pattern of finding is of interest because approximately 40 percent of ulcer patients relapse in the first year after medical treatment. Although there is some evidence that emotional factors such as irritability, anger, and submissiveness play a role in ulcers, their exact role is uncertain; and the involvement of these elements of the AHA! Syndrome in ulcers appears to be not so strong as with problems such as hypertension, heart disease, or cancer.

PUFFING YOUR WORRIES AWAY: SMOKING AND PERSONALITY

Cigarette smoking is thought by many—including the surgeon general—to be the most important preventable cause of death in the United States.[47] Smoking is considered to be the major cause of lung cancer, and it is also a major risk factor for coronary heart disease, arteriosclerotic peripheral vascular disease, chronic bronchitis, emphysema, and cancers of the larynx, oral cavity, esophagus, pancreas, and bladder.[48,49] Over the past two decades, rates of cigarette smoking have declined for both males and females. Current national statistics indicate that about 35 percent of adult males are cigarette smokers while 30 percent of adult females smoke cigarettes on a regular basis. Whereas these trends show a reduction for both males and females, the decline has actually been greater for men because of the higher rates during the 1960s when 50 percent of males were smokers, compared to about 33 percent of females.[50]

It has been reported that up to 80 percent of cigarette smokers who initially succeed at stopping will relapse within a year. Although there are many reasons given for the relapse,[51–53] the most often cited reasons are the experience of significant life stresses—interpersonal problems; relationship problems; job stress—and exaggerated negative emotional responses associated with such events (see Shiffman; Bare and Lichtenstein).[51-53] The stress-coping model of smoking behavior views cigarette smoking as a means of coping. In a general sense, this model assumes that some people turn to smoking because smoking is an effective means of dealing with stressful life events and their consequences. Furthermore, high levels of stress and emotional upset are thought to predispose ex-smokers to relapse, and the smoking is used to decrease negative affect (feelings of anxiety and irritability) and achieve a state of homeostasis or more desirable level of affect. Given this perspective, it could be that smoking also regulates positive affect—increasing positive affect through physiological means or through pre-established associations between smoking and positive situations.

There is indeed ample evidence that stress and the experience of negative emotions associated with stress are related to smoking relapse. However, the factors related to the initiation and maintenance of smoking more often involve the influence of family/sibling/peer smoking habits and certain personality factors related to sensation-seeking. The research literature on smoking and personality is quite diverse and was reviewed by G. M. Smith in 1970.[54] This reviewer observed that smoking has been positively associated with the following personality traits: extraversion (12 of 15 studies); antisocial tendencies (17 of 19 studies); and impulsive behavior (6 of 8 studies). Smith concluded that cigarette smokers are more likely to be extraverted and to have more antisocial tendencies than nonsmokers, and that smokers are also more impulsive and tense. Studies published since the review by Smith have provided further evidence that smoking is associated with extraversion, antisocial tendencies, impulsivity, neuroticism, and anxiety. On the other hand, there appears to be very little evidence that the initiation of smoking is related to elements of the AHA! Syndrome—the major reason being that very few research studies have examined the relationship between cigarette smoking and elements of the AHA! Syndrome.

Although the evidence does exist to support a relationship between smoking and personality factors, there is one major difficulty in interpreting this research data. The problem has to do with the failure to distinguish between factors that influence people to begin to smoke and those that contribute to the maintenance and continuation of smoking once it has been established. One of the most influential studies in attempting to tease out this effect was conducted by my mentor at the University of South Florida, Charles D. Spielberger.[55] This study was reported in 1982 and investigated the relationship between selected personality measures and the initiation and maintenance of smoking behavior. Consistent with previous research, the findings derived from this young adult population showed that smokers score higher than nonsmokers on measures of extroversion, neuroticism, and psychoticism.[55,56] These differences—although in the same direction for both males and females—were stronger for female smokers, who also had higher anxiety scores than nonsmokers, whereas male smokers had lower anxiety scores than nonsmokers. Smoking was found to be unrelated to feelings of anger and irritability. Overall, the pattern of findings from this study led Spielberger to conclude that females, who are higher in neuroticism and anxiety than males, may start smoking as a means to reduce tension and that smoking may be an effective tension reducer for those females who smoke regularly.

Please note that these conclusions are interesting in view of the fact that cigarette smoking and lung cancer have increased significantly among women over the past ten years. This increase in smoking coincides with a time in which there have been substantial changes in the types of stress and frustration that women face in their daily lives as a result of their upward movement in job/careers outside of the home. Among women, cigarette smoking has also been related to other important health outcome factors. For example, a study reported by J. J. Counselman and E. V. MacKay examined smoking habits, baby feeding practices, and a number of personality factors among 1,790 postpartum women.[57] Their findings were, for the most part, in support of previous research showing that cigarette smokers tend to have more emotional problems, more reproductive failures, and babies with lower birth weights than nonsmokers. With regard to baby feeding, smokers tend to have little prior knowledge of breast-feeding and to favor bottle-feeding.

At the University of South Florida, I collected data regarding the relationship between cigarette smoking and the experience and expression of anger; out of this research came my Ph.D. thesis, completed in 1984.[58] In this study, a greater percentage of adolescent girls (33 percent) were cigarette smokers than adolescent boys (22 percent). Smoking rates for white adolescents (35 percent) were also higher than smoking rates for black adolescents (16 percent), with the highest percentage occurring among white adolescent females (41 percent). Although the initiation of cigarette smoking was most strongly influenced by whether an older sibling and the parents smoked, a few measures of anger significantly discriminated between adolescent smokers and nonsmokers. For example, among black adolescents, the frequent experience of intense anger reactions—particularly in situations involving criticism and evaluation—was associated with cigarette smoking. Among white adolescents, the experience of anger seemed unrelated to cigarette smoking. I did discover, however, that the manner in which anger is expressed was related to cigarette smoking in white adolescents. More specifically, white adolescent smokers were more likely to report that they openly express their anger than were nonsmokers.

As we would hope, not all adolescents who start smoking cigarettes continue the habit. In my thesis study, approximately 9–22 percent of the adolescents reported that they were ex-smokers. It was hypothesized that a comparison of the emotional factors discriminating between current smokers from these ex-smokers would provide some information about the role of emotions in the maintenance or continuation of cigarette smoking. Subsequent analyses of the data along these lines showed though that neither of the anger measures discriminated current smokers and ex-smokers among the white adolescents.[59] However, black adolescents who were current smokers reported that they experienced anger more frequently and at a greater intensity—particularly in situations involving time pressures. Thus, it may be that cigarette smoking among black adolescents serves to reduce feelings of anger and irritability.

PSORIASIS AND STRESS

According to Dr. Madhulika Gupta in personal communication with the author, psoriasis is a chronic, relapsing, cutaneous condition with a 1–2-percent prevalence in the general population. The characteristic lesions of psoriasis are erythematous, thickly scaling plaques that can affect any skin area. Overall, psychosocial stress and emotional factors are believed to play a role in the onset or exacerbation of this condition in approximately 40 percent of the persons with psoriasis.

Although there are a number of exceptionally organized studies in this area, very few examine the role of multiple dimensions of stress (e.g., major changes in life circumstances, psychological and emotional factors, and lack of social support from family and close friends) on psoriasis in a single study. For this reason, I have chosen to review here a comprehensive study that attempts to evaluate a wide range of psychosocial parameters among patients with psoriasis. To date, 127 patients with mainly plaque psoriasis have participated in this study, which is being conducted under the direction of Madhulika Gupta at the University of Michigan Medical Center.[60,61] All patients are admitted to the Dermatology Inpatient Unit where they receive a standard course of treatment consisting of topical corticosteroids, anthralin, tar, and ultraviolet-B (UVB) phototherapy. Psychological measures and information about the patients' degree of stress are obtained within the first week of admission to the Dermatology Unit.

One of the stress measures has been used to determine the extent to which patients believe that stressful situations make their psoriasis worse. Basically, those patients who report that stress exacerbates their psoriasis—High Stress Reactors—tend to be more disfigured by the disease as evidenced by greater severity of psoriasis on their scalp, face, neck, forearms, hands, and genital regions—emotionally charged body regions that arouse emotional reactions in patients because of the effect of psoriasis on the patient's appearance and sexuality.

Psychologically, the High Stress Reactors are more interpersonally dependent or tend to rely more on the approval of others, and they report more disease-related stress (e.g., I have to deal with a lot of day-to-day hassles that others don't have to face, because of my psoriasis) in contrast to stress from major life events. On the other hand, patients who report that stressful situations are not likely to make their psoriasis worse—Low Stress Reactions—experience feelings of anger in association with their disease; and the number of daily life stresses they relate to the psoriasis (e.g., other people making insensitive remarks about their appearance; having to avoid certain public places and social situations) is related to its severity.

As indicated above, the degree of interpersonal dependency.or approval from others is strongly related to the severity of psoriasis. Thus, the High Stress Reactors probably fear greater social disapproval as their psoriasis worsens. Furthermore, the tendency of the High Stress Reactors to withhold angry feelings in the face of social disapproval and greater cosmetic disfigurement probably impedes their capacity to cope with the chronic stress associated with their condition. Overall, the study suggests that patients with psoriasis who believe stress makes their psoriasis worse are more likely to have certain personality characteristics such as difficulty with assertion of angry feelings and a tendency to want the approval of others, in addition to more cosmetically disfiguring psoriasis. This personality constellation superimposed on the more disfiguring psoriasis most likely makes such patients more vulnerable to the stresses that result from the impact of psoriasis on quality of life.

Although the mechanisms by which stress and psychological factors may exacerbate psoriasis is currently a matter of speculation, the skin is an important organ for expressing emotion and is the somatic locus of exhibitionism. The most noted examples of emotions expressed by the skin are blushing in shame or embarrassment, and itching as a sign of anxiety, impatience, and irritability. In fact, other research by the team of dermatology investigators at Michigan have revealed that pruritus or itching in psoriasis is strongly related to psychologic symptoms of depression.[61] For example, among a group of 82 patients admitted to the inpatient Dermatology Unit, the degree of depressive psychopathology discriminated between mild, moderate, and severe pruritus groups at admission. After being admitted, all patients received the standard course of treatment, and dermatologic and psychological ratings were obtained for a second time within two days before discharge

Whereas the severity of pruritus was not directly related to the severity of psoriasis, 26 percent (21 out of 82) of the patients rated pruritus as their most bothersome symptom, and more than two-thirds (55 out of 82) reported moderate or severe pruritus associated with their psoriasis. The most salient finding in this study is the significant relationship between the severity of pruritus and the severity of depression at the time of admission. Furthermore, the improvement in pruritus pretreatment to posttreatment was associated with an improvement in depressive symptoms.

5

Fighting and Loving—
Seeing Black and Blue

In 1969, Swiss researcher Max Luscher published a book called The Luscher Color Test in which he describes how colors preference can tell a lot about the personality of an individual.[1] The color test is used widely throughout Europe by psychologists and physicians, and even by personnel managers for screening job applicants. In the United States, a more familiar side of this research has to do with the decorating of certain rooms and the widely held notion that colors can influence our moods, energy level, and health. For example, the walls in the holding cells of many city jails and prisons are medium-pink or light-blue because these are regarded as calming colors. On the other hand, bright yellow is thought to be related to industriousness and overexcitement.

As Luscher sees it, choosing the color blue as the one that is most appealing to you means that you need emotional tranquility, peace, harmony, and contentment in your life. You need your relationships with others to be placid and free from strife. On the other hand, if blue is your least favorite color, you probably have trouble in your relationships with others because they cannot live up to your high standards. If black is your most appealing color, this denotes dissatisfaction with almost everything. You refuse to allow anything to influence your point of view. If black is your least favorite color, you want to be in control of your own actions and decisions.

But what about black and blue? Who would ever show a preference for those awful black-and-blue marks that attest to a chain of events starting in verbal abuse and ending in physically abusive behaviors. Sad to say, those same black-and-blue marks tell much too often of kisses interlaced with punches, and whispers of love and affection traded in for threats. The colors of child and spouse abuse are, without any doubt, deep shades of black and blue. Child abuse and spouse abuse are two of the most extreme forms of family violence. Although the mechanisms by which family violence affects the adjustment of children and parents are poorly understood, the one certainty common to both child and spouse abuse is that the black-and-blue marks of the victims result from poor and inappropriate management of anger-hostility-aggression.

Most of this book deals with the adverse health effects of anger, hostility, and aggression on the individual who experiences chronic and excessive levels of the AHA! Syndrome. However, such strong emotions often arise in the context of interpersonal relationships with important and significant loved ones, such as a child a or spouse. Could it be that angry and hostile people live in environments where there is a high degree of these strong emotions? Are abusive parents simply people who have extremely poor anger-management and conflict-resolution skills? Or do angry, irritable, and poorly socialized children do their utmost to elicit negative behavior and hostile responses from their parents? There is also the issue of spouse abuse and the data suggesting that children who are exposed to violence between their parents are more likely to exhibit both short-term and long-term adjustment problems.[2-9] Retrospective accounts of men who batter their wives indicate an intergenerational pattern of the violence within homes in our society. For example, estimates from a recent national interview sample revealed that sons who witness their fathers' violence have a 1,000-percent higher rate of wife abuse than sons who do not.[6] Is this simply a case of the son's modeling the father's approach to managing conflict?

Although upsetting to consider in their full extent, these problems are a part of life in modern times, and the roots of both child and spouse abuse are deeply embedded within the AHA! Syndrome.

THE ROLE OF ANGER IN CHILD ABUSE

The mistreatment and harsh physical punishment of children has been sanctioned throughout history, often in relationship to cultural norms for disciplining and educating children, pleasing certain gods, or expelling evil spirits. Furthermore, until the nineteenth century, these acts were condoned and supported by law, and often considered salutary. Public interest and awareness of the incidence and severity of child abuse has changed dramatically over the past decade. For example, Time magazine reported that in 1976 only 10 percent of the U. S. population considered child abuse to be a serious national problem, whereas a recent Louis Harris survey revealed that the concern has risen to 90 percent. However, according to psychologist David Wolfe at the University of Western Ontario, the manner by which the public has been made aware of child abuse may represent an unfortunate roadblock to the understanding and prevention of child abuse.[3] In other words, the successful campaigns stirred up by the communication media have created a public image of the abusive parent as a seriously disturbed individual. Documentary films, too—such as <u>Mary Jane Harper Cried Last Night</u>—have helped to shock the public and lawmakers into realizing the extent of the problem. Whereas the general public views the abusive parent as being grossly aberrant and psychologically unfit, the consensus among researchers is that only approximately 5 percent of abusive parents exhibit such extreme symptomatology.[3,8] According to Wolfe, this perceptual discrepancy may seriously limit research on the causes and consequences of child abuse, as well as efforts to prevent this problem.

Incidence of child abuse

Information it had gathered on the incidence of child abuse led the National Center on Child Abuse and Neglect to estimate recently that 351,000 children (5.7 per 1,000) are physically (inflicting bruises, cuts, burns, or internally injuries due to non-accidental behavior), sexually (exposing a minor under the age of 18 to sexual acts or materials), or emotionally (insulting or berating the child) abused by their caregivers each year.[10] Less conservative estimates of the extent of this problem were reported in 1980 by M. Straus and associates.[2,6,11] The Straus estimates—based on extrapolated data from a representative nationwide survey—indicate that between 1.4 and 1.9 million children each year receive serious injury from a family member. Also in 1980, the American Humane Association reported that there are nearly 800,000 cases of child maltreatment in this country.[12] Therefore, regardless of the variability among estimates, the rates of child abuse are alarmingly high. Compared to all U.S. families with children, maltreated children are twice as likely to live in a single-parent, female-headed household; they are four times as likely to be supported by public assistance; and they are affected by numerous family stress factors such as health problems among parents, alcohol abuse, and spouse abuse.

One important fact about the incidence of child abuse that is not often emphasized is that its victims—particularly those who are seriously abused and injured—are extremely young: The average age of child abuse victims is 7.2 years, and the average age for those who die as a result of their injuries is 3.3 years.[12] In many of these cases, the parents have repeatedly injured their children. But if so, then why are these cases not detected earlier? Part of the answer may lie in the fact that definitions of abuse vary widely from one community to another and from one group of public health workers to another. Also, the case that many types of injuries that result from abuse are difficult to detect or to classify. And those parents who repeatedly injure their children may take them to different hospitals or doctors in order to prevent the injury of the child from being classified as abuse rather than of accident.

Estimates regarding the long-term consequences of child abuse are difficult to calculate. However, child abuse has been implicated in the etiology of serious antisocial behavior occurring later in life, and in the perpetuation of family violence through generations. For example, according to J. D. Alfaro, an average of 50 percent of the families reported for child abuse in New York State have had at least one child who was later taken to court for delinquency or being ungoverned.[7] As David Wolfe and other psychologists have suggested, a child who is exposed to the use of violence as a conflict resolution technique may fail to develop adequate means of coping with anger, hostility, aggression, and the tension related to stressful life situations.[3] Therefore, child abuse is a concern not only because of the immediate physical and psychological harm to the child, but also because it may have a traumatic impact on the child's future behavior. I would add that the victims of child abuse who do not develop effective means of coping with anger-hostility may be more susceptible to the onset of major health problems over the long run, as well as interpersonal difficulties.

Background Characteristics of Abusive Parents

Interest in the child abuser's psychological functioning has been intense over the past two decades, although this interest has produced no consensus with regard to distinctive personality attributes or serious emotional disturbances among abusive parents. As indicated earlier, the perception of the abusive parent as a seriously disturbed individual may be due in part to the clinical impressions reported in the first decade of research, and to the successful media campaign that publicized the extent of the problem. Whereas abusive parents rarely show severe psychological disturbance, professional opinion in the 1970s—as reported by John Spinetta and David Rigler—converged on the general assumption that child-abusive parents have a defect in personality, allowing aggressive and hostile impulses to be expressed too freely.[8] These reports also suggest the presence of inadequate and poor impulse control, an immature personality, and antisocial personality characteristics. Recent studies comparing abusive and nonabusive parents have challenged these earlier assumptions, however. Today most researchers view child abuse as a learned pattern of maladaptive behavior, rather than a psychiatric disorder. According to David Wolfe, for instance, inadequate behavior patterns that are situation specific—such as dealing with aversive child behavior (e.g., child who never stops crying or clinging for attention), problem solving with other family members, and handling chronic levels of emotional stress—appear to define the abusive parents more accurately.[3]

A determination of the child abuser's psychological characteristics is extremely difficult because of the different methodologies used to measure underlying personality attributes or traits. For the most part, the comparability of findings from one study to the next is questionable. However, a recent review by Wolfe of empirical studies on the child-abusive parent attempted to overcome certain of these difficulties.[3] Overall, there were 20 studies that met the selection criteria for being included in the review. These criteria were: (1) a definition of the child abuse sample indicating that the parents and children were under the supervision of a child protection agency due to alleged or confirmed physical abuse; (2) observational or self-report measures having known or reported psychometric properties, being valid and reliable; (3) a research design that controlled for major demographic factors such as education and income levels of the parents; and (4) a complete presentation of results enabling the reviewers to evaluate and interpret the findings.

Basically, Wolfe's review indicated that studies using measures of deep-seated personality abnormalities have been unable to detect any patterns associated with child abuse beyond general descriptions of "displeasure in the parenting role" and "stress-related complaints." Overall, the majority of studies fail to find significant differences between abusive parents and normal control parents on multiple measures of personality functioning. However, there are two studies that found more self-reports of psychological ill-health symptoms among abusive parents. Interestingly, both studies found abusive parents to report more anger, unhappiness, rigidity, and inflexibility with regard to the parenting role, compared to nonabusive parents. There are also a number of investigations that have found elevated reports of affective and somatic distress among abusive parents. For example, a study reported by R. Conger and associates revealed that abusive parents are more likely to have physical health problems than nonabusive parents.[5] This finding was interpreted as being related to the fact that the abusive families in the study experienced more negative life changes than the nonabusive families.

Several recent investigations have also found child-abusive parents to have more symptoms of depression as well as more physical and emotional distress than nonabusive control groups.[3] And a few studies suggest that the increase in psychologic distress is related to negative interactions between the abusive parent and the children.[4,5,8] In other words, when child-rearing is stressful—as in the greater occurrence of negative life changes among abusive families—there may be an increase in signs of emotional and somatic distress. Moreover, the parental ability to use nonabusive disciplinary skills may be strongly influenced both by the degree of emotional stress related to family-mediated events and by somatic or physical health problems. I would add that the somatic complaints and health problems may be partially related to the greater occurrence of life stress, as well as the parents' poor management of anger–hostility. It is also possible that child-abusive parents have an enormous difficulty dealing with their negative emotional reactions to unpleasant or aversive social events in general. That is, abusive parents may not be subjected to any more stress than nonabusive parents; they may simply perceive their environment to be more stressful, aversive, and debilitating than nonabusive parents do. To a certain extent, the data reviewed by Wolfe lend support to this opinion.

In the area of child abuse, anger and hostility often surface against a background of increased psychosocial stress. As discussed in earlier chapters, the AHA! Syndrome of Anger–Hostility–Aggression is often associated with specific stressful events or challenging circumstances, especially in the case of individuals who are characterized as manifesting strong Type-A behavioral traits (see Chapter 3, particularly). This is also true for child-abusive parents, since a confrontation between the parent and the child over disciplinary issues is the context of most child abuse.

In the vast majority of child abuse cases, the parents are ineffective and inconsistent in their use of discipline, and the children who are abused tend to present parents with more disciplinary problems than do children who are not abused. Unfortunately, most parents face the task of caring for young children under less than ideal circumstances. Many of the abusive parents have little financial security, are young and in the process of learning to work together, and are still in the process of making their own transition from adolescence to adulthood.[3,8,11] These stresses while at the same time raising a child can place a tremendous psychological, social, and economic burden on parents. Furthermore, it is becoming more common for the hardship of child-rearing to be faced by single parents. In 1960, nearly 10 percent of all children (6 million kids) under the age of 18 years old resided in one-parent families. The number of children living in this situation doubled between 1960 and 1978 and the figures have increased again between 1978 and today.

Given the forever-growing inflation and unemployment rates, it is little wonder that the psychological distress—depression, cynicism, anxiety—related to these stressors has become worse, or that the frequent and intense experience of anger and hostility has reached such an exceedingly high level in our society.

Some Triggers of Child Abuse

It has been argued that the majority of child abuse occurs in the context of confrontations between the parent and child over discipline.[12-15] If this be true, then what determines the escalation of irritable and angry behaviors among certain parents and not among others? Are there certain behaviors exhibited by the child that elicit these angry episodes and lead to abuse? Could it be that certain parents have a stronger disposition to experience feelings of anger in response to stress and have severe problems with their verbal and behavioral expression of anger? Certain psychologists—Kenneth Dodge and colleagues, for instance, provide a convincing case for the possibility that individuals with a strong disposition to experience anger, hostility, and aggression often make misattributions about the behaviors of other people with whom they are interacting.[9] Behavior viewed by others as neutral may be perceived by an aggressive–hostile parent or child as indicative of hostile intention, and therefore becomes part of the sequence of events that leads to episodes of anger, irritability, and conflict. Problems of this nature are complicated further by the fact that people interacting with aggressive and hostile individuals also make misattributions. In one study in this area, psychologist Gerald Patterson reported the likelihood to be .040 that an aggressive boy with discipline problems would initiate coercive behaviors, given that the mother was behaving in a neutral or prosocial fashion.[13] The comparable likelihood for an aggressive–hostile mother acting in a coercive manner was .047 when the child had been behaving prosocially or neutrally. As it stands, however—unlikely as they are—these "surprise attacks" would contribute to the overall uncertainty in problem families, and contribute to the frequent experience of anger and irritability that escalates into nasty and abusive confrontations between parent and child.

Be that as it may, well-behaved children in normal and non-distressed families also present their parents with many occasions for discipline. For example, P. Chamberlain reported that among 85 families who were nondistressed in terms of child–parent relationships, almost two-thirds revealed they had at least one child-management problem that was chronic.[14] The most commonly reported problems, in descending order, were: (1) arguing, (2) defiance, (3) noncompliance, (4) talking back, (5) whining, and (6) complaining.

While the major focus in child-abuse prevention research is on high-risk families with young children, poor management of aggression and hostility is generally indicated by an excess prevalence of overt anger expression in the home, as well as by a general acceptance of corporal punishment as a proper form of discipline. It has been estimated that more than 90 percent of parents in this country either consistently use or occasionally resort to spanking and other types of physical coercion to resolve disciplinary problems. In a study of 2,000 parents by R. J. Gelles, nearly 20 percent had pushed, grabbed, or shoved their child more than twice during the previous year—while almost 10 percent had kicked, bitten, or hit their child with a fist or other object more than twice.[11]

As indicated earlier, the initiation and maintenance of disciplinary issues are involved in most instances of child abuse. As shown by Gerald Patterson and his colleagues at the Oregon Social Learning Center, much of the irritable behavior of both abusive and nonabusive parents is in reaction to the abrasive behavior of a poorly socialized child.[13,15] The thing that separates the child-abusive parent from the nonabusive—parent, according to research by John Reid and Kate Kavanagh—is that child-abusive parents tend to become more irritable and angry.[16] A 1983 study by John Reid showed that mothers from a sample of distressed families rated their daily discipline confrontation as significantly more angry than did mothers of "normal" families who were not experiencing child–parent relationship problems.[17] In this study, the mothers described their previous day's discipline confrontations, and rated each one on a seven-point scale (1 = not angry; 7 = furious). The average scores for the mothers from distressed families with abused children was 3.5, which was significantly higher than the rating of 2.5 for the mothers from nondistressed families.

Other important research findings from the Oregon Social Learning Center are based on the assessment of negative affect in natural settings. Over the past 5–10 years, the group of psychologists and researchers at Oregon have made considerable progress in devising methods for observing and coding social interaction in the home. For example, observer judgment about shifts from neutral affect to positive or hostile affect is based on changes in facial expression and voice or tonal inflections. Negative affect—described as a general disposition to react in an angry, irritable, and hostile manner to others—is measured by duration in seconds during family observation periods. Recent data reported by Gerald Patterson showed that, among normal families, 80–90 percent of the interactions were characterized by neutral affect and that most of the recorded shifts from neutral affect tended to be positive rather than negative.[13] For the most part, negative affect and facial expressions, and increases in tonal inflections or voice changes, occurred at a low frequency and lasted briefly for mothers of normal, non-distressed families. On the other hand, mothers from distressed families with problem children exhibited negative affect more frequently and for longer periods of time during the observation sessions.

To check on the validity of the observational assessment the anger and hostility scores of the mothers as obtained from a questionnaire and the observer's "global" rating of negative affect as determined immediately after the session (before the video-recorded interaction session was coded and rated) were compared to the ratings of negative affect during the session. As expected, there were modest correlations between the anger–hostility scores (and the observer's global affect ratings) and negative affect exhibited during the family interactions. Furthermore, mothers who exhibited a high level of negative affect during the observation sessions were more likely to counterattack when the child initiated a deviant action. Most importantly, these mothers were more likely to persist in being irritable. No matter how the target child responded—neutral, or even in a positive fashion—the mother was geared for a fight.

One other finding that deserves to be mentioned is that those mothers who were at the extreme for negative affect during the observation sessions also tended to be at the extreme for irritable content. In other words, those mothers who frequently react to their child with negative affect also tend to express and display more feelings of irritability and anger. Overall, the pattern of findings from this study suggests that strong and intense maternal negative affect is more strongly related to the maintenance and continuation of conflict than to the start of a conflict.

In addition to the stresses of child-rearing, research implicates other stressors in triggering anger episodes and conflict as related to child abuse. For example, compared to nondistressed families, families with severe child-management problems have fewer positive contacts with people in the community (supportive friends and family members; people to turn to in times of trouble), and more negative contacts; and the negative contacts are typically initiated from outside the family. This may in fact help to explain why abusive families—while not subjected to significantly more negative life changes and socioeconomic disadvantages than nondistressed families—perceive their life circumstances to be more adverse and debilitating. Interestingly enough, several well-constructed studies have shown that these perceptions of adverse environmental and family conditions are strongly associated with the failure of abusive parents to seek out and use available support and resources in their communities. Marital conflict has also been shown to be associated with child abuse.[3,11,16] In addition, social factors such as family structure, education, age at birth of first child, and situational and financial stress on the family have been implicated.[18] As indicated earlier in this discussion, emotional problems such as negative affective states and depressed mood of parents are associated with a decreased ability to cope with discipline situations and lead to an increase in faulty judgments or misattributions about the behavior of the child.

In a 1987 study, Susan Crockenberg at the University of California–Davis Campus examined the predictors and correlates of anger toward and punitive control of toddlers by adolescent mothers.[19] In this study, the impact of rejection and acceptance experienced during the adolescent mother's childhood, social support received after the baby's birth, infant irritability, and angry outbursts were examined. Possible links between such maternal behavior and the child's anger and noncompliance, low confidence, and social withdrawal were also investigated in a sample that included 40 mothers who had given birth as adolescents and their 2-year-old children. Basically, Crockenberg's findings showed that adolescent mothers who had experienced rejection during childhood and received little support from a partner after the child's birth were more likely to exhibit angry and punitive parenting behaviors. On the other hand, infant irritability did not predict maternal behavior.

Of equal if not more importance, the results showed that angry and punitive mothers tended to have children who were angry and noncompliant and who distanced themselves from their mothers. Most importantly, among angry and punitive mothers the occurrence of infant irritability as early as three months postpartum was a strong predictor that the toddle would be angry and noncompliant. The early occurrence of infant irritability also predicted those infants who exhibited less confidence at 2 years of age. These findings clearly support the notion that there is a reciprocal relationship between angry and punitive maternal behavior and the degree to which the infant is irritable and difficult to manage. At least for a 2-year-old child, it would appear that the level of anger and noncompliance is dependent on the coexistence of both factors: punitive maternal behaviors, and early infant irritability.

Interestingly enough, the pattern of results discussed above tends to generalize across cultures. For example, similar findings were reported by A. Engfer and K. A. Schneewind, who investigated the causes and consequences of harsh punishment in a representative sample of 570 German families.[20] Furthermore, the conditions that predicted harsh parental punishment are, in the rank order of their importance: (1) a child perceived as difficult to handle (a problem child); (2) parental anger-proneness; (3) rigid assertion of parental power; and (4) intrafamilial problems and conflicts. Personality problems of the child basically included a wide range of conduct disorders and emotional problems such as excessive irritability and anger, anxiety, depression, and helplessness.

Apparently then, most incidents of child abuse involve a great deal more than the use of corporal punishment with a child during a coercive battle. As the parent (and the child) loses control and accelerates from low- to high-intensity punitive and aggressive behaviors, the potential for physical injury to the child—who is often quite young—increases. In the case of child abuse, the situational cues involved in the transition from anger to hostility and aggression often involve aversive behaviors on the part of the child, as well as the parent's poor skills in coping with the conflicts and anger that often center around disciplinary actions.

Explaining how anger may lead to excessive aggression, Leonard Berkowitz maintains that the paired association of aversive and noxious events (such as the child's arguing and talking back to the parent, or child tantrums) with otherwise neutral stimuli (such as the child's laugh or certain facial expressions) may evoke angry, hostile, and aggressive behavior from the parent during subsequent parent–child interactions. Presumably, the parent is responding to cues that have been associated previously with strong feelings of anger and frustration, and the parent's reactions toward the child may be in part determined by this conditioning.

According to Berkowitz's this model, then, child-abusive parents would be expected to exhibit an enhanced emotional arousal—as reflected by physiological responses—to events and situations that resemble stressful situations they have encountered previously. As it turns out, a small number of highly organized studies do clearly show that physiological response patterns obtained from abusive parents are more enhanced and reflect greater emotional arousal than similar measurements obtained from nondistressed families. Although most of these data were based on the parents' responses to videotaped portrayals of parent–child conflict, the studies generally validated the situations as stressful (or nonstressful) by having the parents rate the situations. Taken together, these findings suggest the possibility of a hyperarousal–anger–abusive behavior pattern. In other words, when a parent exhibits heightened physiologically mediated arousal in the presence of negative and aversive child behaviors, that parent may be prone to respond with irritable and angry behaviors. Also, that parent may become less capable of utilizing appropriate strategies for managing conflict and anger, and more capable of abusive acts that would never happen were she or he more physiologically cool.

Psychosocial Impact of Abuse

Although a discussion of the impact on the child of various types of abuse and neglect is beyond the scope of this book, I do feel a need to give at least my impression of the extent of the problem. As I say, this is an impression—one gained by reading and crying my way through many disturbing research reports on the topic. In general, verbal abuse and sexual abuse have a greater impact (than physical abuse) on children's perceptions of themselves and the environment in which they live. Such children are more angry and pessimistic about the future. Also they do not believe that the abuse (verbal or sexual) is their fault. However, physically abused children appear to be more accepting of the blame for being mistreated—at least when the mistreatment is mild or moderate, but not when severe.

Across the many studies, there is also a tendency for the physically abused children to report feeling that they were unwanted at birth. And in fact, there are a few studies that show a relationship between the extent that the mother wanted her child and the extent of abuse. As a group, children who are abused have more developmental delays in language, self-control, and peer interaction. Studies of abused elementary-school children (and younger children) show that they often have significant learning and motivational problems at school, as well as a higher rate of aggressive and destructive behavior. Finally, studies of abused children who have somehow managed to live to reach adolescence show that they are more likely to engage in juvenile crime, commit violent offenses, and have alcoholic and criminal parents than nonabused adolescents.

Given the poor management of anger-hostility among abusive parents, one may well wonder if the quality of their health is any worse than that of nonabusive parents. Although abusive parents generally do not exhibit symptoms of severe psychological disturbances any more than nonabusive parents, they are prone to a wide range of stress-related disorders such as depression and health problems. In the long run, these health problems are likely to impair their ability to cope with the stressful demands of parenting. However, although in most cases the health problems of abusive parents are thought to be related to stress, it is quite possible that the angry and hostile family environment is itself the root of the health problems . At least I want to believe that. In this regard, a prospective study reported by R. W. Levenson and J. M. Gottman provides evidence of one possible physiologic pathway whereby chronically abrasive and stressful relationships might influence immune system functioning and increase the susceptibility for health problems.[22] This study showed that greater autonomic arousal in interacting married couples is strongly predictive of a subsequent decline in marital satisfaction and an increase in marital stress. More importantly, poorer health ratings at a 3-year follow-up were strongly related to greater declines in marital satisfaction.

Given that unhappily married persons report poorer health than either divorced or happily married persons, then it is possible that the persistent physiological arousal associated with a disturbed and problematic relationship could lead to alterations in endocrine and immune functioning, and might increase the risk for becoming physically ill. Although this is part of the explanation for the association between suppressed hostility and mortality among the husbands and wives in the Tecumseh Community Health Study (see Chapter 1),[23] the exact pathway between suppressed hostility and mortality is still unpaved and awaits future research.

DOES TALKING ABOUT ANGER GET IT OUT OF YOUR SYSTEM?

COUPLE GETS INTO ARGUMENT ABOUT "TEMPER SURVEY"!

A township couple completing a magazine questionnaire on "How Fast Does Your Temper Flare Up?" found out a few days ago, and neighbors called the police. Troopers responded to a call about 10 a.m. reporting a domestic dispute at a local apartment complex. At the residence, troopers found the couple in a heated argument over the article. The pair promised to calm down, and one of them told troopers she was moving out.

Although we can't really tell whether this couple learned how fast their tempers flare up, I would bet they did learn that talking about anger is not the way to get it out of your system. In fact, there tends to be a positive reciprocal relationship connecting one's outward expression of anger and both an increase in the intensity of one's own anger as well as the possibility of provoking anger in the other person. Many readers of this book may have figured it would say that it is always beneficial to express anger openly. This belief is very prevalent among psychotherapists and the general public. But actually, in most cases it is terribly difficult to discuss anger openly because of the shouting, crying, threats, screaming, and physical assaults that often accompany revealed anger. Although the debate as to whether the discharge of feelings—or catharsis—is beneficial has a long history (see Chapter 1 for a brief account), research shows that venting anger and hostility in reaction to a provocation does not usually help people to feel better. Carol Tavris, a social psychologist and author of the book Anger: The Misunderstood Emotion, revealed that, when people express anger in a hostile or aggressive manner, they do not get rid of it at all.[24] In fact, people who are likely to vent their feelings of anger tend to get angrier—not less angry. Instead of feeling good after expressing anger, most people feel miserable, sad, irritated, depressed, guilty, and shameful, and some people wind up in physical pain or covered with black-and-blue marks as a result of physical assaults linked with the open expression of anger.

Now, I am not saying that the way to deal with angry and hostile feelings is to suppress them and keep quiet. On the contrary, unexpressed anger can cripple people emotionally—leaving them with strong feelings of depression, anxiety, guilt, and frustration. The tendency to suppress anger—much like the tendency to have a short temper—is learned in relationships. Parents teach their children that many negative feelings—especially anger—are undesirable. When either the suppression (Anger-In) or the expression (Anger-Out) of anger is used rigidly and consistently to the extreme, it becomes a habitual way of coping and dealing with anger; and both ways of coping can be psychologically damaging. For example, one of my recent studies of more than 500 young adults showed that individuals with elevated Anger-In scores as well as those with elevated Anger-Out scores have more symptoms of depression and anxiety, and score higher on measures reflective of a more frequent and intense experience of anger and hostility than their counterparts with lower levels of Anger-In or Anger-Out.[25]

So it appears that one of the keys to the effective management of anger is to express anger, yes, but in appropriate ways that address whatever is triggering the emotion. Most psychologists believe that anger can be a highly constructive tool, serving as an alarm that something is wrong in our relationships with others—or whatever—and thus providing the impetus to change whatever is triggering the emotion. There is no doubt that discussing anger can lead to practical solutions to the things that are wrong in one's life, but one's perception of the causes of anger as well as one's state of physiological arousal can be strongly affected by the very act of talking about the causes and consequences of anger. As in the case of some child-abusive parents, the reason that talking out anger does not reduce it is that talking out the anger is often associatively paired with noxious events (such as yelling, screaming, threats), increased physiological arousal, and otherwise neutral situations (such as a child's or spouse's facial expression) that can evoke these angry and hostile reactions in subsequent interactions. Presumably, the individual who spends time talking out anger episodes that are related to personal problems is not getting rid of the anger, but is—as Carol Tavris says—"practicing it" or going through a rehearsal of just how angry and furious she or he really is about the situation triggering the emotion.

It would appear, then, that having people talk about important life events that are both stressful and associated with intense angry episodes would elicit strong physiological and emotional reactions. Furthermore, if individuals with high blood pressure and hypertension have problematic ways of coping with and expressing anger, then their physiological reactions should be more exaggerated than individuals with normal blood pressure. These hypothesis are the focus of my current research on the psychological and behavioral factors related to hypertension in young adults. In order to conduct these studies, a highly sensitive interview referred to as the Structured Anger Assessment Interview (SAAI) was developed. Because the questions comprising the SAAI are structured (i.e., always in the same order), it has been possible to gather information with a high degree of comparability about the physiological responses related to talking about anger over a wide range of life events (problems with job, marriage, family, finances, etc.). The SAAI was developed to measure various dimensions of the experience and expression of anger, and to elicit verbal and behavioral manifestations of anger and hostility. Because the SAAI is an audiotaped (or videotaped) psychological-challenge interview, the answers to the questions can be rated for their specific content, and a verbal–behavioral assessment can be conducted on the general stylistics and mannerisms of the subjects as they answer the questions.

In many ways the SAAI is similar to the Structured Interview developed by Drs. Ray Rosenman and Meyer Friedman for assessing Type-A behavior (see Chapter 3).[27] Although my research with the SAAI is still in progress, some of the results as displayed in Figure 5-1 show that the systolic (SBP) and diastolic (DBP) blood pressure readings and the heart-rate (HR) responses of young men with borderline hypertension (BT) are significantly higher than those of their counterparts with normal (NT) blood pressure.[28] Interestingly enough, the men with borderline-hypertension were more expressive, spoke in a louder tone of voice, focused more on themselves as reflected by their greater usage of personal pronouns (I, me, my, mine), and exhibited a strong potential for hostility (more use of sarcasm, profanity, and rude statements) during the SAAI. The findings with regard to self-references are remarkably similar to an earlier study by psychologist Larry Sherwitz of the University of California at San Francisco.[28] In his study, blood pressure responses to a stressful laboratory task were larger for subjects who used more self-references.

In the SAAI, once the interview has been completed, the men rate the level of irritability, annoyance, and anxiety they experienced during it. Although the men with mild hypertension experience greater levels of physiological arousal and exhibit a strong potential for hostility, their ratings of irritability and annoyance during the SAAI have turned out to be no different from the men with normal blood pressure. It seems that—for

Figure 5-1
Cardiovascular responses of borderline and normotensive during Anger interview

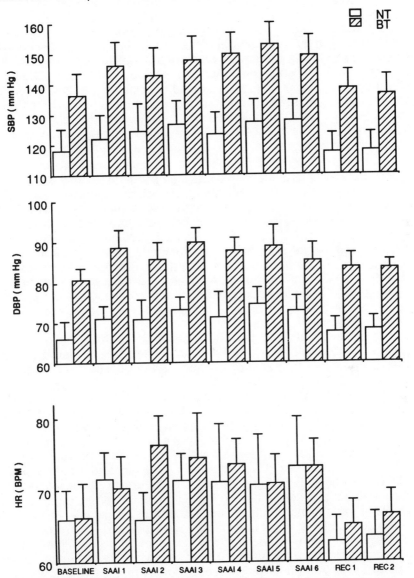

Source: Derived from Johnson, E.H. Cardiovascular reactivity during Structured Anger Assessment in black males (abstract). <u>Psychosomatic Medicine</u> 1989, 51:244.

whatever reasons—men with borderline hypertension have a stronger disposition to experience anger and hostility as well as heightened cardiovascular arousal, but have difficulty identifying and labelling their feelings.

Perhaps these findings suggest that some people—hypertensives, in particular—have difficulty with their perception of bodily sensations and feedback from others. If we assume that the interview was presented in a challenging manner and was devoid of feedback about the appropriateness of any response, then it must be that the content of the answers caused the rise in blood pressure. Similarly, studies conducted by Joel Dimsdale and his colleagues at the University of California in San Diego showed that the blood pressure response to a stress interview was greater for hypertensive patients, compared to normotensive control subjects.[30] The interview used in Dimsdale's research amounts to an intense discussion about areas in the subject's life that are currently stressful rather than pointed questions about the subject's experience of anger–hostility related to stressful events in general. Nevertheless, the stress interview led to large increases in blood pressure for the hypertensives. As Figure 5-2 demonstrates, the blood pressure responses elicited by the interview were higher for both hypertensives and normotensives than those elicited by two standard laboratory tasks (the first, a mathematical calculation complicated by superimposing a loudly ticking metronome; the second, a cold pressor test in which the subject is required to place his or her foot in a pail of cold water for 90 seconds).

If the emotions and the physiological arousal we experience in relation to stress are related to environmental cues and feedback from others, then how an interviewer presents the questions about anger should have some influence on the intensity of the anger being discussed. This is precisely the research issue that was investigated by Ebbe Ebbeson, Birt Duncan, and Vladimir Konecni in the mid-1970s among aerospace-defense employees (mostly engineers) who were about to be laid-off. The timing of the notice for the layoffs was such that it came after one year, rather than at the end of the three-year contract that had been promised to the employees. Therefore, the workers had a right to be upset and angry. In order to determine if the content of present verbal aggression has an impact on future verbal aggression, a sample of more than 100 employees underwent an exit interview where the questions about anger and hostility were directed either toward the company (Are there aspects of the company you don't like?), their supervisor (Are there things about your supervisor that you don't like?), or themselves (Are there things about yourself that led your end of the exit interview, the employees completed a report telling what they thought about the layoff. Results from this unique study showed that the employees who became most angry and hostile toward the company or the supervisors during the exit interview were also those who blamed the company and the supervisors in the written report. On the other hand,

Figure 5-2
Average systolic/diastolic blood pressure during seated baseline, mathematical calculations, cold pressor test, and stress interview

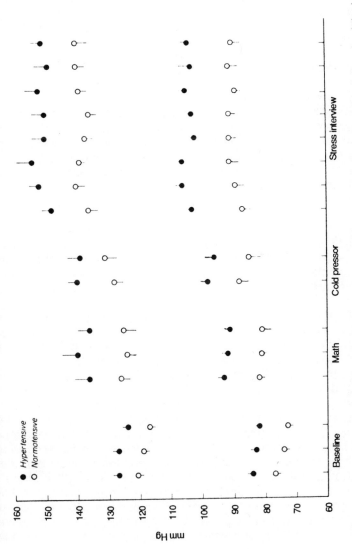

Source: Dimsdale J.E., Stern M.J. and Dillon E., The stress interview as a tool for examining physiological reactivity. Reprinted with permission from <u>Psychosomatic Medicine</u> 1988, 50:68.

the employees who blamed themselves did not get so angry as those employees who were angry at the company or the supervisors.

In a related study, psychologist Prudence Brown—while working with Ernest Harburg at the University of Michigan—wanted to know whether the manner by which women coped with and expressed anger had any impact on their psychological well-being when going through a divorce.[32,33] Brown interviewed 253 women as they registered at a marriage counseling service that was court related, and again after four months. The findings from this most extraordinary study revealed that women who expressed their anger outwardly did not differ from women who suppressed their feelings of anger related to the divorce. There was essentially no difference in the level of psychological distress, anxiety, depression, and self-esteem. However, when Brown compared the women who had felt an improvement in their psychological well-being over the four months with those women who remained unhappy and depressed, she discovered that the improved women talked less obsessively about the divorce.

Another way of thinking about these findings is that the women who had a strong attachment to their ex-husbands had a difficult time disconnecting or detaching their emotions and themselves from the disturbing events related to the divorce or separation from their husbands. Anger is a strong sign of deep attachment and connection with an important or significant individual. In the case of separating couples going through the process of a divorce, anger is rarely used as a constructive tool to change whatever is wrong with the relationship or the behavior of the spouses. On the contrary, anger tends to be the catalyst that initiates the divorce, formulates the legal settlement, and fuels the heated arguments. However, as discussed in Chapter 4, the feelings of anger and negative attachment to the spouse that are often associated with this stressful time appear to have a bad impact on the disease process.

To summarize, then, talking about anger—or talking out anger—is one of the best ways to stay angry and intensify other bad feelings. During anger episodes—or the blind rage—some people probably suffer a breakdown in their ability to perceive appropriately and label their feelings, physical sensations, and bodily responses. Individuals may be angry and disturbed about certain facets of their life but not even realize that they sound, look, and behave angrily. Chronically angry and hostile individuals often have social skill deficiencies that result in a lack of sensitivity to interpersonal problems and feedback from important people in their lives. It is often the case that angry individuals fail to consider the possible consequences of their behavior, and for the most part they are unable to see the provoking situation from the perspective of the other persons involved. If the attribution of blame for these angry and hostile interactions as recalled and reinforced during talks about the anger with friends and associates is projected onto others, then the feelings of anger will probably become more intense. It is also my belief that talking out anger will result in anger being experienced for a longer duration and could possibly erode into hostility, fighting, threats of violence, and other aggressive behaviors. In other words, there may be much truth to the ancient Chinese proverb, "The fire you kindle for your enemy often burns you more than him."

SPOUSE ABUSE—WHEN LOVE HURTS

As indicated earlier in this chapter, the one common denominator associated with child abuse and spouse abuse is that the victim suffers from the culprit's inability to cope appropriately with and manage feelings of anger. There is a very firm link between abusive behavior and other forms of family conflict. For example, Murray Straus's summary of interviews conducted within a nationwide sample of 1,146 persons who were living with a partner and children revealed that previous exposure to harsh physical abuse as a child and to marital violence and disharmony as an adult are significantly associated with higher rates of severe violence toward children.[34] According to Straus, the explanation for this association is related to the fact that violence in one sphere of life tends to carry over into other spheres. In general, these interviews also showed that mothers are more likely to use physical punishment with children than fathers, and that the degree of violence toward a child is associated with marital violence—more so for women than for men. Several exceptional studies in this area have revealed that abusive parents emit a higher rate of aversive behaviors (yelling, threats, arguments) toward their spouses and other family members than nondistressed or nonabusive families.[3,6,8,11]

Several retrospective studies of men who abuse and batter their wives indicate that the vast majority have witnessed similar behavior on the part of their fathers.[6,11] Estimates from a nationwide sample suggest that sons who witnessed their fathers' violence have a 1,000 percent greater rate of wife abuse than sons who did not. Furthermore, there is a growing body of evidence showing that wives are less likely to seek refuge from their abusive husbands if they witnessed their mothers being the victims of spouse abuse.[11,34,35] The statistics also show that domestic violence cuts across race and class lines. In any case, estimates are difficult to calculate because of a lack of knowledge about the various forms of abuse and the fact that most victims remain silent and do not report the incident. Moreover, the battered woman has not been a clearly recognizable presence to medical caregivers, and victims rarely report abuse to the primary care provider without being asked.

Data on marital violence are hard to come by, as people are often reluctant to disclose what they feel is an embarrassing, shameful and private parts of their lives.Although the national survey reported by Straus shows that husbands and wives are about equally abusive to each other (see Table 5-1)[34,] these data have been severely criticized by other investigators who believe that wives are more likely to be abused than husbands.

As to the characteristics of spouse-abuse victims, the impression I have formed after reading the diverse literature in this area is that the victim has low self-esteem and intense feelings of anger and hatred that have been internalized because of the consequences related to their outward expression. In many victimized women, this leads to self-destructive behaviors such as alcohol or drug abuse. Although many of the victims' behaviors are predictable and best understood in the context of learned helplessness, there is no particular personality pattern that leads one to become a victim of abuse. Rather, in general, women are often socialized to be submissive; and in the process, those who are likely to become victims of abuse may not develop adequate self-protection skills as children, especially if they come from families where the mother was abused. Basically, the men who are usually the culprits of spouse abuse have been socialized to express strong negative feelings of anger and hostility. Often these men have learned to model the abuse witnessed or experienced in childhood; and consequently, women are

Table 5-1
Use of Force at Least Once within the Past 12 Months among Married Couples in the United States

Type of Force	Husbands	Wives
1. Threw something at spouse	2.8%	5.2%
2. Pushed, grabbed, shoved spouse	10.7%	8.3%
3. Slapped spouse	5.1%	4.6%
4. Kicked, bit, or hit with fist	2.4%	3.1%
5. Hit or tried to hit with something	2.2%	3.0%
6. Beat up spouse	1.1%	.66
7. Threatened with knife or gun	.4%	.6%
8. Used knife or gun	.3%	.2%

Source: Adapted from Straus,M. A. Wife-beating: How common and why? In Straus, M. A. and Hotaling, G. T. (eds.), The Social Causes of Husband–Wife Violence. Minneapolis: University of Minnesota Press, 1980.

often the recipients of their physical violence. Although a number of different theories are used to explain the causes of marital violence, several of them link marital violence to power. In other words, if a man's dominance and achievements are strongly valued in the society and culture, then his achievements outside of the home (at work) establish his dominance and power in the home. But, when the guy is considered or considers himself a failure, he resorts to violence and abuse to maintain dominance and control in the marriage.

Marital violence occurs more often when the couple is under stress from events such as unemployment, financial difficulties, or pregnancy. Abusive couples are also extremely isolated; they do not have many friends, and their ties with relatives are not strong. In many instances, the loss of supportive bonds with family and friends acts both as a cause and as an effect of marital violence. That is, being isolated may increase stress and provoke abuse, but having an abusive and violent marriage may lead to withdrawal from contacts with friends and family.[36]

The notion of "learned helplessness" is often used to explain battered women's coping responses to their partners' abusive behavior, or why a woman would choose to remain with her batterer. However, a number of other reasons have also been given for why battered women stay entrapped in severely abusive relationships. Some have to do with economics: She feels that on her salary alone she cannot meet the financial responsibilities of the house, the kids, or the lifestyle she has come to enjoy therefore, she cannot afford to leave him. Other reasons are based on psychosocial factors: She does not want the children to grow up without their father in the home; she thinks that a violent father image is better for the children than no father at all. Still, other reasons are less tangible and relate to the abuser's ability to make the victim think that his low opinion of her is correct, and his ability to make her believe that they are powerless and stuck in a situation that is unchangeable. As several researchers have suggested, women involved in abusive relationships seem to have problem-solving deficits that interfere with their ability to actualize effective solutions to problems. Researchers Margaret Launius and Bernard Jensen examined this hypothesis by studying a group of women who had been battered and a control group of nonbattered women.[35] The women who had been in a battering relationship gave evidence of deficits in several skills necessary for solving problems. In essence, the battered women perceived fewer options, generated fewer plans, and chose fewer effective solutions in both abusive and nonabusive problem situations. These results were taken to mean that battered women have a generalized problem-solving deficit, rather than faulty cognitive perceptions that are specific to their handling of the abusive relationship.

For some women, it is difficult to escape from an abusive relationship because escaping means letting go of the love they feel for their man as well as letting go of the tormentor. The basic problem here may be that the love a woman brings to a relationship is much more complete, deeper, and more involved than that of most men. I am not saying that men are not capable of cultivating deep feelings of love, but that it hurts women more to give up on love and disconnect the link between their feelings and the object of their love. Unfortunately, many women choose to remain in abusive relationships long after the love that they cultivated and nourished has become physically, verbally, emotionally, or sexually abusive. As indicated above, there are many reasons for a woman's choosing to remain with her batterer; but the most painful reason, in my opinion, is love—when the relationship is killing her.

HOW DOES ALCOHOL CONTRIBUTE TO THE ANGER PROBLEM?

Large amounts of alcohol act as a depressant, while alcohol in small amounts is a stimulant. As with any substance taken into the body, there is probably an "optimal" or moderate level of alcohol intake that does not disrupt the homeostatic balance of the body and mind. The problem with alcohol is that it is often used while we are socializing and celebrating accomplishments or happy occasions as well as when we feel down-and-out. What makes alcohol so appealing is the very thing that contributes to its being so dangerous: Its ability to loosen conversation, let people forget their worries, and allow them to doing things they normally would not do. It frees impulses and behaviors by impairing second thoughts. So, it would appear that small amounts of alcohol may act as a social lubricant by stimulating and bringing life to a party, but too much can result in individuals becoming depressed, cynical, bitter, and angry.

Alcohol is probably the most commonly used drug in the United States, and it sometimes leads to antisocial behaviors and reactions in people who—when sober—exhibit no violent, hostile, or aggressive tendencies. Given that so much family violence occurs in the context of excessive alcohol usage, one of the consequences of alcohol—apparently—is to intensify negative feelings and emotions that are related to stressful and problematic interpersonal situations. Thus, when individuals drink to forget about stressful problems in their life, they may start talking about their situation, become more intensely angered or feel less inhibited, and then allow those feelings of anger to escalate into hostile and violent behaviors. In these instances, the alcohol distorts the ability to think straight and pinpoint the causes of personal difficulties. This can result in excessive behavior ranging from increased aggressiveness to a total disregard about one's personal safety or the safety of others as in drunk driving. Research on violent crimes such as stabbing and homicides has shown that alcohol was a factor in 64–88 percent of the cases studied.[37,38] Similarly, the antisocial behavior of many juvenile delinquents is associated with problem drinking,[39] and research by Selzer and associates suggests that the high proportion of intoxicated drivers involved in fatal traffic accidents may be in part a reflection of the effect of alcohol on aggression and hostility.[40,41] For these reasons, numerous theorists in this area have suggested that alcohol serves as a stimulator or releaser of aggressive behaviors.[42–45]

In fact, several well-organized laboratory studies have demonstrated that alcohol consumption is predictive of increased aggressive behavior even among social drinkers. For example, Lang and colleagues studied the effects of alcohol on aggressive behavior in male social drinkers.[45] Half of these subjects were led to believe that they would be drinking alcohol (vodka and tonic), while half believed that they would be drinking only tonic. Within each of these two groups, half of the subjects actually received alcohol, while half were given only tonic water. Following administration of the beverage, half the subjects were provoked to aggress by exposing them to insults from a confederate of the study. Aggression was measured by the intensity and duration of shocks administered to the confederate on a modified Buss aggression apparatus. As it turned out, regardless of the actual alcohol content of their drink, subjects who believed they had consumed alcohol were more aggressive than subjects who believed they had consumed only tonic water.

Despite considerable research on the effects of alcohol on behavior and psychological well-being, there is very little information about its influence on interpersonal behavior and judgment regarding human emotions. In one of the few studies in this area, Josephine Borrill, Bernard Rosen, and Angela Summerfield tested the hypothesis that alcohol would affect an individual's ability to judge facial expressions of emotions.[45] To test this hypothesis, 30 male and 30 female normal social drinkers were given either a high level of alcohol, a low level of alcohol, or a placebo and were then shown photographs of faces displaying basic emotions. The subjects who consumed the high level of alcohol made more errors than subjects in the low-alcohol condition, who made fewer errors than subjects given the placebo. Although the accuracy of judgment varied significantly according to the sex of the subject (males made more errors than females), alcohol was associated with greater impairment of judgments when in came to anger than to any other emotions. From this it should be clear—only if you are not drinking—that mixing anger with alcohol results in a diminished ability to use anger in a constructive manner.

Since anger is a transactional response that involves feelings, bodily reactions, perceptions, and reactions from others, alcohol's effects make it difficult to address the problem that is triggering the emotion. In this regard, individuals who find themselves in heated arguments after having too much to drink are not only frustrated and upset about their failure to pinpoint causes of the anger; they are also engaging in the very behaviors (talking out anger, yelling at each other, etc.) that intensify and prolong the experience of anger—which could lead to violence.

Isabel Birnbaum, Thomas Taylor, and Elizabeth Parker measured the relationship between alcohol consumption in 93 women social drinkers and their mood and cognitive efficiency both while they were sober and after consuming alcohol.[47] In this group of women, a strong relationship was found between alcohol consumption and self-reported feelings of anger and depression while the women were sober. In a second examination six weeks later, women who had reduced their alcohol intake were more likely to have decreased their anger, depression, and mental confusion when they were sober, relative to women who maintained or increased their alcohol intake.

Most people do not want a messy argument or fight. Yet when angry, resentful, and a bit intoxicated, they easily build up steam for a brawl when others fail to see their point of view. Maybe if the intoxicated person did feel listened to, some of that anger and resentment might not be overtly manifested.

The major conclusion I would draw from this brief review of the relationship between alcohol and anger is that the consumption of alcohol can serve as a catalyst for intensely felt anger and rage. Alcohol is not the only cause of family violence, but it helps to set the stage for an enormous amount of the violence and abuse that occurs between spouses or partners and between parents and their children. Alcohol probably plays so large a role in family violence because it impairs thinking and impulse control. As a consequence, some individuals who are able to control and manage feelings of anger and hostility when sober—by recognizing the consequences of their behavior, and because they do feel listened to—are not capable of controlling strong aggressive impulses when under the influence of alcohol.

6

Gender and Ethnic Differences in the Experience and Expression of Anger

The basic impression that most psychologists have about gender and ethnic differences in anger is that men and members of minority groups are more likely to experience intense feelings of anger and resentment. Men are expected to express anger openly, while women are supposed to feel more depressed and suppress their anger because they are afraid to express it and because it is unladylike to "lose your temper." Men, on the other hand are encouraged to express their feelings of anger because it is part of the achievement-oriented, aggressive, macho, and masculine role image that is reinforced in our society. It is as if a man's worth in our society were viewed by his achievements while a woman's value were judged by the successfulness of her relationships. In the not so distant past, self-esteem was evaluated in terms of one's fulfillment of roles that were tied to strong gender stereotypes. For a man, his worth and value to himself and his family depended on his occupation, his job, his earnings. For a woman, her survival was seen as dependent on her relationships—particularly the success of her marriage. In the context of these stereotypes, when a man lost his fortune he lost his pride, self-respect, and confidence in his ability to cope with life. Precisely the same process is believed to occur in women who lose important love relationships. For both men and women, the losses are thought to result in depression and low self-esteem. And although these image and self-worth differences are based on strong sex-role stereotypes, many of us—some more strongly than others—believe that they do influence how males and females cope with stress and frustration.

Developmental studies, for example, indicate that there are gender differences in both the traits developed and the time of their occurrence.[1,2] Interestingly enough, boys are more likely to be aggressive and belligerent at every stage, and their psychomotor skills develop earlier while their cognitive and language capacity lags behind girls. Furthermore, a large amount of information has been gained about the role of male and female anger in interrelationships from observations of children while they are playing. During play activities, boys are more aggressive—constantly yelling, arguing, and fighting. No matter how rough or how violent the activities become—playing continues and goes on. Girls, on the other hand, will bring play to a halt if things become too rough. In many such instances, the girls refuse to continue playing; they simply walk away from the situation. Moreover, it appears as if girls will do their most to preserve the friendship and relationship with their playmates, while boys are consumed by a passionate desire to beat each other up or chase each other until someone is declared the winner. Are these differences the roots of a gender difference in the experience and expression of anger?

Black people and other members of disadvantaged minority groups in the United States are presumed to have special difficulty expressing their anger directly and effectively. Supposedly, blacks assume a passive-aggressive attitude and act sarcastically—as women tend to do—rather than express feelings of anger and irritability in an open and direct manner. In the case of women, venting their anger openly, directly, and loudly gives the impression of being unfeminine, unladylike, or sexually unattractive.

For blacks, the simple truth may be that feelings of anger and irritation are not expressed openly because of the fear of retaliation and counterattack. In many instances, the root of this fear is quite real. One need only think about the level of joblessness and the job turnover among young black men to understand why they tend to suppress rather than express anger.

One young well-educated black woman who participated in our studies on the physiological responses to anger provocation revealed that she does not get angry when treated unfairly, but instead she "gets even" and does not bother to be nice then about what she is saying or the manner she uses. In fact, many of the women who have participated in our studies report that they do not have difficulty expressing anger and irritability—the same is true for young black males and females. However, there are a few common threads that weave through most gender and ethnic study groups. Most of the time, the self-reported frequency of anger is quite low; and most people report that they do not manage or express anger very well.

Another common thread is that the cause of anger is generally due to the frustration associated with thwarted plans. For example, in an early study among college students—reported by Ann Anastasia and colleagues—approximately 52 percent of the anger responses were due to thwarted plans—with the interfering agent consisting of individuals or institutional factors, in the majority of cases.[3] The next most frequently aggravating stimuli were situations causing inferiority and the loss of self-esteem and prestige.

WHICH SEX HAS THE PROBLEM WITH ANGER?

To begin with, few studies have been conducted directly to examine gender differences in the experience and expression of anger. The lack of research on this topic and the failure to question the belief that men are more prone to experience anger than women is like assuming simply that the women who stay in bad relationships love too much and the men do not love enough. In any event, the truth of the matter is that the connection between anger and gender is not simple. For example, research methods to determine how or why people experience anger and how this troubling emotion is expressed, suppressed, and controlled often vary from study to study. Some researchers rely on the psychological testing techniques that derive data from responses to questionnaires, while others gather information by asking people questions about real and recent experiences. For the most part, anger—like other emotions—is not a discrete and static event that involves a single stimulus and single response. Anger is a complex emotional response that includes elements of past injustices and provocations, along with a desire to change the behavior of the culprit. Anger also involves the expression of frustration and dislike for the object of the anger episode, and the experience of a wide variety of emotions (guilt, shame, rage, embarrassment, depression) before, during and following the anger.

Because the word "anger" is so often used interchangeably to describe hostility and aggression, it does not take much stretching of the imagination to see why males would be perceived culturally as more likely than females to behave in an aggressive and angry manner when faced with threat and provocation. And researchers are now beginning to gather convincing scientific data that support this notion. [4-7] Studies of human males and nonhuman primate males suggest that there may be a positive relationship between testosterone levels in adolescence and adulthood, and certain forms of aggressive behavior.[4-8] However, a positive relationship is not necessarily a causal linkage. In this case, the relationship between testosterone and aggression may be a function of other factors that were not considered.

Researchers in Norway, however, did take the time to make a convincing test of the hypothesis that testosterone influences aggressive behavior. In this study, Dan Olweus and his colleagues selected 58 healthy boys of 15–17 years old from the public school district of Solna, of Stockholm Sweden.[8] The boys completed a number of personality inventories, including measures of verbal and physical aggression. Peer ratings provided information about each boy's habitual level of aggressive behavior (e.g., starts fights; verbal aggression against teachers; unprovoked verbal aggression against peers). In addition to these variables, detailed information about the boys' temperamental characteristics and rearing conditions during childhood had been obtained from their mothers and fathers when the boys were 13 years old. The basic findings of this study suggest that circulating levels of testosterone in the blood plasma have a direct causal influence on provoked aggressive behavior. High levels of testosterone also lead to an increased readiness to respond vigorously and assertively to provocations and threats. In the study, high levels of testosterone made the boys more impatient and irritable, which in turn increased their propensity to engage in aggressive-destructive behavior.

Several studies have examined the relationship between testosterone and criminal violence among prison inmates. For example, James Dabbs and colleagues determined that inmates with the highest testosterone concentrations had more often been convicted of violent crimes.[9] The relationship between testosterone and violence was most notable at the extremes of the testosterone distribution—where 9 out of the 11 inmates with the lowest testosterone levels had committed nonviolent crimes, and 10 out of the 11 inmates with the highest levels had committed violent crimes. Interestingly, among those inmates convicted of nonviolent crimes, those with the highest testosterone levels received longer terms to serve before parole and longer punishments for disciplinary infractions (generally assaultive behavior)s while in prison. Overall, the average testosterone level for inmates rated by their peers as "tough" were no different from those rated as "weak." Actually, testosterone was related to peer ratings of toughness, but only among inmates living within the weaker dormitories. The "weaker" dormitories were described in the study report as less intense and wild, and the researchers believed that the peer ratings could have been more reliable for men living in the weaker and calmer dorms. In any event, testosterone was highest only among those inmates in the weaker dorms who were rated as tougher by their peers.

Although there appears to be fairly good evidence then, for a hormonal basis of aggressive behavior in males, the findings from the available studies on this topic do not preclude the possibility that early learning experiences are important determinants of aggressive behavior in both males and females.

Adolescents and Anger

My own research on the differences in anger between males and females was stimulated by several findings revealed in my Ph.D. thesis.[10] As part of the post-doctoral project, information about the experience and expression of anger was derived from questionnaires administered to 601 male and 459 female adolescents. I found some differences between males and females in their disposition or trait to experience feelings of anger and irritation.[11,12] However, to my surprise, adolescent females had somewhat higher trait-anger/temperament scores than adolescent males. This finding indicates that, at least among adolescents, females have a stronger tendency to experience intense feelings of anger more frequently—particularly in situations where they feel they are being evaluated unfairly or threatened. Adolescent males, on the other hand, scored significantly higher than females on psychological measures indicating that they react with more intense angry reactions when they are pressured by time and deadlines. The overall pattern of these findings indicated that adolescent males and females do differ in their likelihood to experience anger, and these differences are dependent on the social situation that is the stimulus and cause of the provocation.

In this study, the adolescents also completed several questionnaire measures of anger expression. Neither sex had any great difficulty expressing anger outwardly at objects or other people. In other words, male and female adolescents did not differ in their likelihood of doing things like slamming doors, throwing things, being nasty, making sarcastic remarks, or arguing with others. However, the two sexes were different in their likelihood of suppressing anger and irritability. Adolescent males were more likely than females to do things like pout or sulk, harbor grudges, withdraw from people, be angrier than willing to admit, at the time, and feel irritation a great deal more than the people in their environment realized. Further analysis of the differences between males and females revealed that, regardless of gender, adolescents with a high level of suppressed anger were more likely to report experiencing strong anxiety and fear about expressing their anger.

On the other hand, it was discovered that the frequent outward expression of anger was determined mainly by the frequency with which anger itself was experienced. Again, our findings were similar for adolescent males and females. As might be expected from the evidence on catharsis mentioned in Chapter 5, the aftermath of an angry episode leaves a sour taste for both adolescent males and females. Both groups reported a considerable amount of guilt following the expression of anger, and the adolescent males were just as likely to feel guilt as were the adolescent females.

Recently we conducted a follow-up investigation of the relationship between suppressed anger and anxiety/fear among adolescents.[13] This new study included a number of important psychosocial factors relevant to anxiety such as: (1) level of psychological disturbance, (2) amount of social contact with friends, (3) satisfaction with social contacts among family and friends, (4) availability of family and friends for support when faced with a crisis, (5) sleeping disturbances, and (6) somatic symptoms. Although males scored higher than females on suppressed anger, there were no differences between the sexes in the relationships between suppressed anger and the psychosocial factors. In other words, both male and female adolescents with high levels of suppressed anger (e.g., pouting and sulking; withdrawing from people; being angrier than willing to admit) were more anxious and psychologically disturbed, experienced more stressful life events, reported more sleeping disturbances and somatic complaints, and had fewer family members and close friends available for support in a crisis . In a similar study, Judith Siegel found that adolescents who get angry quite often tend to be overweight, relatively sedentary at school and on the job, and more likely to be characterized as Type-A.[14] Adolescents who frequently experience anger that is directed outward tend to be anxious, have elevated blood pressure, and are relatively sedentary during leisure time. Smoking, the occurrence of negative life events, and low self-esteem are associated with both the frequent experience of anger in many social situations and the outward expression of anger. Interestingly enough, these findings were maintained after controlling for both gender and age (all respondents being 13–18 years of age). In other words, the pattern of these findings is similar for males and females.

So, what clear conclusions can be drawn about gender differences in the experience and expression of anger among adolescents? First of all, there are a few strong and consistent differences that appear to depend on the social situations associated with the provocation. For adolescent males, these social situations tend to involve the stress and frustration of time pressures; for females, the situations are more likely to include unfair evaluation and threat. Second, adolescent males are more likely than females to suppress their feelings of anger, while both sexes are similar in the degree to which anger is expressed outwardly at other people and objects in the environment. There is also good evidence that testosterone has an important role in aggressive behavior among males, but early learning experiences are also undoubtedly important determinants of aggressive behavior. For example, several recent studies of chronic adolescent offenders—both males and females—apprehended for assaultive crimes have revealed that, when parents tolerate violence in the home, this acceptance of hostility and aggression is generalized by the adolescent to outside the home as a method of resolving interpersonal and social conflicts.[5,6,8] Third and finally, there is some evidence that destructive associations between anger and behaviors detrimental to good health (e.g., smoking, elevated blood pressure, psychological stress, sedentary lifestyle, Type-A behavior, inadequate social ties with family and close friends) are found in adolescents. Although it is not possible to predict whether that the interrelationships between anger and these risk factors will contribute to poor health, it is my opinion that the management of anger needs to be targeted for modification early in life.

Young Adults and Anger

Are the differences in anger for adolescents consistent for other age groups? Basically, the answer to this question is a qualified no. According to data accumulated by Charles D. Spielberger, there are few strong differences between the experience and expression of anger for college students and other young adult groups.[15] Surprisingly, females tend to score slightly higher than males on measures of the disposition to experience strong feelings of anger, and young adult females score slightly higher than males on suppressed anger: but the differences are not large enough to be significant.

My research findings on gender differences in anger among young adults are based on data obtained in 1988–1990 from 300 male and 300 female (age 18–35-year-olds) residents of a small town in Michigan. These respondents are the young adult offspring of residents who participated in the Tecumseh Community Health Study (see Chapter 1). In this study, young adult females did not differ from males in either the expression or the aftereffects—feelings of guilt—of anger. However, the women were more likely to experience strong feelings of anger and anxiety frequently, as well as report a higher level of fear and anxiety about expressing anger. Men in this study were more cynical, bitter, and dominant than women.

So it appears that some subtle differences in anger arise between adult males and females. Interestingly enough, the overall pattern of our findings for young adults in Tecumseh, Michigan, is remarkably similar to data recently reported by B. S. McCann and colleagues.[16] In their study of 97 male and 111 female undergraduate college students, women scored significantly higher than men on anger-emotionality and guilt, resentment, and irritability—but lower on assaultiveness and anger expression. In other words, the women reported that they experience feelings of anger and irritation more frequently, but they tend not to openly express these feelings or engage in aggressive and resentful behaviors. If anything can be concluded about the relationship between anger and gender, then, it would have to be that women report they experience anger more often—and not less often—than men, and yet women do not generally show it.

The Differences between Men and Women

When contradiction occurs in the direction of the results, one must question whether it is a function of the research methods. Personally, I believe that the differences in perception between men and women—although subtle and difficult to follow—are true and that a great deal of our difficulty in sorting out the real truth about anger and gender is inherently related to how well we researchers ask our questions. Fortunately, researchers have used various methods to assess anger. In one study, psychologists Douglas Frost and James Averill recruited a large sample of men and women (age 21–60 years) and interviewed them about recent experiences of anger.[17] All participants responded to questions about some real anger episode that had occurred within the previous week. Unlike the questionnaire measures of anger, the findings derived from this interview of adults revealed very few differences between men and women. For example:

1.   Causes of Anger—Both men and women were most likely to have
      gotten angry at (1) someone they love (spouse, lover, parents);
      and then, (2) situations that involved an arbitrary violation of their
      rights and expectations; and then (3) someone who attacked their
      self-worth and self-esteem, or someone who had wrongly eval-
      uated their performance.

2.   Angry Reactions—Both men and women reported feeling entitled
      to express their anger because the person(s) involved in the anger
      episode was well aware of what he or she (or they) was doing, and
      had no right to do it. Thus, men and women apparently justify their
      reactions in the same way when they feel angry. The majority of
      men and women (58 percent) reported that they had expressed
      their anger outwardly, while 13 percent reacted aggressively (hit-
      ting, slapping, throwing things, slamming doors). Both men and
      women were similar in the degree to which they would take their
      anger out on a third person or object, talk to the target of the provo-
      cation, or try to calm themselves down in private.

3.   After Effect of Anger—There were essentially no differences in the
      degree of guilt, shame, and embarrassment experienced by men
      and women following anger episodes. Approximately two-thirds of
      the men and women also said they felt hostile and aggravated,
      while about 50 percent felt depressed, anxious, and nervous
      following the recent provocation. About a third of the group said
      they felt relieved and satisfied about expressing their anger. In fact,
      both men and women cited the same reasons for expressing
      anger: to change the behavior of the target; to assert authority; to
      strengthen the relationship with the target of the provocation; or to
      let off steam and express dislike. More women than men said they
      were likely to cry when they felt anger, and to deny the object of
      their anger some customary benefit such as a nice home cooked
      meal.

      To gain additional insight into the perception of anger among
women and men, I conducted a survey in November 1988. It was not so
complicated as the one by Frost and Averill, but the findings were quite
interesting. There was no attempt made to secure a random sample; the
participants were very diverse in their ages (25–48 years old),
occupations (secretaries, laboratory technicians, physicians, nurses,
biostatisticians, psychologists), and races or ethnic origin (white, black,
Asian). A total of 50 individuals (25 men and 25 women) were
interviewed. The questions in the interview focused on four areas: (1)
the causes of anger; (2) the reactions during anger episodes; (3) the
aftereffects of anger; and (4) crying after anger episodes. Basically, all
respondents were asked whether they think men and women are

different or similar on these four points. The results of this survey are as follows:

1. Causes of Anger—seventy-six percent of the women thought that men and women are angered by different reasons, while 44 percent of the men agreed with this opinion. The women said they were most often angered by negative, unfair, and condescending treatment, while angry feelings in men were attributed mostly to verbal and physical challenges—mostly from other men.

2. Reactions during Anger Episodes—Eighty-eight percent of the women thought that men and women differ in their reactions (both verbal and behavioral), while 76 percent of the men agreed with this opinion. Overall, more women thought that men are less likely to verbalize their feelings and thoughts and that men are more likely to behave aggressively (throwing things, verbalizing more threats, slamming doors) and rudely (saying nasty things) while angry.

3. After-effects of Anger—sixty-four percent of the women said that men and women differ in their emotional reactions (guilt, shame, sadness, embarrassment) following anger episodes, while 68 percent of the men believed this to be true. The overall outcome was that both men and women thought women are more likely to feel feel guilt, shame, depression, and embarrassment following anger episodes.

4. Crying—Eighty-eight percent of the women thought that men and women are different when it comes to crying after an anger episode, with women being more likely to cry; 80 percent of the men men thought that women are more likely to cry during and following anger episodes.

What conclusion can be drawn from this brief study? Basically, men and women agree that there are differences between men and women in the aftereffects of anger: Women are more likely to feel guilty, gloomy, sad, and so forth; and women are more likely than men to cry during and after episodes of anger. Furthermore, when one considers the causes of anger, women are more likely than men to say that the causes of anger are different for men and women. Could it be that these perceived differences in the causes of anger have deep roots in the socialization process that encourages males to be more aggressive and to focus on "winning" and achieving more and more in less and less time? It may be that the men and women participating in this survey do really believe—still—that men are more likely to become angry and hostile when there is a threat to their occupational status and personal career achievements, while women are more likely to become enraged when their relationships with significant others are threatened. So why is there such a great gap in the ratio of men to women regarding the perceived causes of anger? I am not sure. But nonetheless, it would seem that the majority of these modern-day women think the causes of anger are different for men and women, while the majority of men think they are similar.

To a certain extent, differences in the perception of anger for women and men may be related to a hypothesis derived from the research of psychologist James Averill, suggesting that people with stronger norms against aggression will account for their own angry feelings and aggression by interpreting it as passion—that is, as being the result of an external cause and due to uncontrollable circumstances.[18] In this context, women—who are generally believed to have stronger norms against aggression and hostility—would be expected to account for angry feelings and aggression by perceiving an angry provocation as being externally caused and uncontrollable more so than men would. In a recent study to examine this hypothesis, M. Egerton had a group of women and men evaluate an angry incident as if they had taken part in it themselves.[19] Overall, the women picked out more conflict in the angry episode than the men did, but the women had a low consensus in using "passion" schemes to explain the angry episode. On the other hand, the men had high consensus in using passion schemes. In other words, men (more so than women) with strong norms against angry aggression were more likely to interpret the angry episode as externally caused and uncontrollable. In another condition where the protagonist wept, there was a greater consensus among the women in using a passion scheme to explain the episode, but no consensus among the men. Overall, the results obtained in this study suggest that sex role has an important effect on the appropriateness of the strategy used to explain angry aggression episodes.

Perhaps, as discussed earlier, people perceive the catalyst for self-esteem and self-worth of men and women as originating from different places. The worth of a man might be more strongly tied to his occupation, achievements, and "public image"—the image that others have of him—while a woman's worth may be strongly linked to the integrity of her relationships. These findings do not suggest that one sex has a greater problem with anger than the other; they simply indicate that men and women differ in their perceptions of the causes of anger.

Interestingly enough, the majority of the men and women who participated in the survey that I conducted agreed that there are differences between the verbal and behavioral reactions of men and women during anger episodes. Within this small sample of well-educated, upper-middle-class and females, the word was that men are less likely to talk about their feelings and thoughts while angry, and that men are more likely to talk and behave aggressively and rudely during anger episodes. However, it is quite possible that elements in the social context of the provocation may contribute to a higher expression of anger among males. For example, if there is any truth to the notion that the sources of self-worth, self-esteem, and pride are attributable to different processes for men and women, then perhaps a man is more likely to express and show anger when provoked in a public place—where there is a threat to his public image—or when confronted by a person of authority such as an angry boss.

These are some of the issues that psychologist Don Fritz attempted to deal with in his research on anger in men and women in real-life situations.[20] Overall, Fritz found very few differences between men and women in their likelihood to experience and express or suppress feelings of anger. However, he discovered that the location of the anger episode (at work, at home, in public) is one of the most important factors determining how men and women act and behave when they are angry. For example, in public places, women are as likely as men to feel angry when provoked or treated rudely, but men are more likely than women to express their anger openly or use their anger to do something to change the situation. The story about anger in the work environment is quite different, however.

Although both men and women cited work as the location in which feelings of anger and irritability are most often experienced, the sexes did not differ in the degree to which anger was expressed at work. These findings are similar to, but a little at odds with, those of Ernest Harburg. In his random sample of men and women living in Detroit, the majority of the working-class men said that they would protest directly to an unjust and angry boss and also report the boss to the union. Although there was no difference between men and women in these reactions, women were more likely than men to be reflective in their encounters with an angry and unjust boss. In other words, women were more likely to bypass the anger and focus on a problem solving approach to the provocation by talking to the boss about the episode at a later time. Not only does it seem that this approach to dealing with anger in the work place would produce less stress, but also findings by Harburg and his associates showed that adults who respond to an angry boss with reflection have lower blood pressures than individuals who use other anger-coping styles.

By now, you are probably as confused as I am about whether the anger problem is worse for men or women. The conclusion I have formed is that both sexes have trouble with the management and expression of anger, and that there are probably some subtle but important differences in how men and women react and communicate while angry. As for gender differences in the experience of anger, I am one of those men who agree with the 76 percent of surveyed women who said that the causes and reasons for anger episodes are different for men and women. I am not sure of all the reasons for this, but I do feel that as more and more women, entering the work place they are being confronted with many of the same stresses and frustrations that men face, and this may ultimately change how both women and men deal with anger.

It is even possible that the pressures on the modern-day working woman are of a magnitude far greater than those on her male counterpart, who does not have her multiple pressures of being a career woman, mother, and wife. Women are likely to develop a conflict between the traditional ideal of nurturance and the importance of family relationships on the one hand and the desires for independence, achievement, mastery, and current female sex-role ideals on the other. I would think that the woman working outside the home must experience a great degree of emotional distress—guilt, anxiety, anger, shame—over this conflict.

Derived from all of the data I have examined, my opinion on the question of gender differences in anger is best summarized in terms of what goes on when males and females are discovering each other—the mating game. I could talk about how little boys and girls deal with frustrations while they are playing. Instead, I will begin with the mating-game of the human adolescent male, who is probably more likely to suppress or hold in feelings of anger than his female friend. Perhaps he is simply trying to do his utmost to show her that a relationship with her is important. Maybe this young male has holstered his six-shooter and is now ready to seek and win her approval. He is still aggressive, but his feelings of anger are more easily stirred in situations involving the pressures of time; while the adolescent female does not like to be evaluated unfairly and is likely to become enraged by condescending treatment from both males and females. And then there is the hormone—testosterone—and its possible impact on the experience and expression of aggression and anger.

During late adolescence and the college-age years there appears to be a more even temperament between males and females. Both sexes are probably busy trying to figure out life and make major career decisions. However, there is a gradual souring of good intentions during young adulthood. If the findings derived from our sample of residents in Michigan are correct, then women are more prone to identify negative feelings as anger. Neither sex has any difficulty expressing feelings of anger; but men are more cynical and bitter, while women are more anxious and fearful about expressing feelings of anger.

Could it be that some women are fearful of expressing anger because this outward display of assertiveness could lead to further negative feelings and problems in her relationship? On the other hand, might some women be afraid to express anger simply because, in the past, it has led to physical aggressiveness and violent actions? Based on a report of some 72 studies of adult aggression that was prepared by Ann Frodi, Jacqueline Mcaulay, and Pauline Thome,[22] I would have to say that women are anxious and fearful about expressing their anger for both of these reasons. However, given the divorce rates and the number of single parent households headed by a woman, it may very well be that women are more anxious about the potential loss of a love object and source of economic support. The report by Frodi and her associates showed that husbands and wives are not different from each other with regard to the likelihood of direct physical aggression when angry. For example, a national sample of 2,143 U. S. families revealed that 12 percent of husbands and wives had attacked each other physically within the past year.[23] In half of these families, both spouses attacked each other at about the same frequency, while the husband was abusive in one-fourth of the cases and the wife was abusive in one-fourth as well. The effects of abusive attacks, however, were worse when men attacked women.

I am still baffled about the differences between men and women concerning the causes of anger. As I said earlier, I agree with the 76 percent of the women and the 44 percent of the men who believe that the causes of anger are different for men and women. However, I would qualify my opinion because I think that these differences are partly related to something more basic: the problems of communicating. Carol Tavris sums this up nicely:

> Problems of communicating are built into the very language habits that men and women have. Imagine this situation: a man and a woman meet at a cocktail party and are attracted to each other. They chat for twenty minutes or so, and as they do their mutual attraction fades. Although they have been talking about shared concerns—the miserable subways, good Italian restaurants, Woody Allen—he walks off thinking she is a chattering intrusive nitwit and she walks off thinking he is an arrogant chauvinist brute.
>
> What went wrong? They may search for reasons for their reciprocal irritation without hitting on the mere subtle one: a clash of conversation rules. When females talk to females, they might ask more questions, fill more silence, and insert more frequent "um-hums" and murmurs than men do. When males talk to males both parties tend to regard any interruption as a challenge to the speaker, who may yield his turn or speak louder to maintain it. When females talk to males, their respective language rules can create misunderstanding. He takes her supportive murmurs as a sign of agreement rather than attention, and feels irritated by her interruptions. She wonders why he isn't paying attention to her and never seems to support what she is saying. When women talk to women in natural settings, for example, they interrupt each other with equal frequency. When men and women talk, men overwhelmingly interrupt women. Women generally respond to male intrusions on their speech by yielding the floor, or by taking longer to reply (as if they were waiting to see if the conversational ball were truly in their court), or by leaving sentences and thoughts unfinished.(Tavris 1984, pp. 201–2).[24]

The difficulty men and women have in talking to each other is widely recognized. Most people have at some time experienced the pervasive sense of despair and hopelessness associated with attempts at "connecting" and "getting through" to the opposite sex. Given that the differences in conversation rules are problematic enough, there appear to be gender differences in self-disclosure as well. It has frequently been found that women self-disclose more than men, but this difference depends on the type of information that is being disclosed. For example, Z. Rubin's study of self-disclosure patterns among dating couples in the Boston Couples Study revealed that females disclose information that is personal and feelings oriented, and may involve negative emotions such as anger, irritability, and depression.[25] Males, on the other hand, disclose more than females about information that is factual (e.g., political views) and very neutral or nonemotional. The trouble that men and women have in communicating is made more difficult because women are more sensitive to social and nonverbal cues, better listeners, and more likely to empathize with the speaker's feelings. On the other hand, women are more likely to show strong negative emotions during interpersonal conflict and send more double messages in their communication. Such behavior makes it difficult for us guys to know what's going on.

Could it be that this difference in conversation rules is the catalyst that influences women and men in their differing perceptions of the causes of anger? And is the difference in conversation rules also the reason a woman can become angry at a man without his having the foggiest idea why?

My answer to these questions is yes! It is easy to think of many situations where miscommunication could lead to some serious misunderstanding that would result in two persons becoming intensely angry. In Appendix C, I have included a couple of questionnaires to complete if you want to see the similarities and differences in how you and your spouse express feelings of anger.

BORN BLACK AND SEEING RED: THE PSYCHOLOGICAL DILEMMA OF BLACK AMERICANS

The facts, however obfuscated, are simple. Since the demise of slavery, black people have been expendable in a cruel and impatient land. The damage done to black people has been beyond reckoning. Now are we beginning to since the bridle placed on black children by a nation which does not want them to grow into mature human beings. The most idealistic social reformer of our times, Martin Luther King, was not slain by one man; his murder grew out of that large body of violent bigotry

America has always nurtured—that body of thinking which screams for the blood of the radical, or the conservative, or the villain, or the saint. To the extent that he stood in the way of bigotry, his life was in jeopardy, his saintly persuasion notwithstanding. To the extent that he was black and was calling America to account, his days were numbered by the nation he sought to save. Black men, however, have been so hurt in their manhood that they are now unsure and uneasy as they teach their sons to be men. Women have been so humiliated and used that they may regard womanhood as a curse and flee from it. Black men have stood so long in such peculiar jeopardy in America that a black norm has developed—a suspiciousness of one's environment which is necessary for survival. Black people, to a degree that approaches paranoia, must be ever alert to danger from their white fellow citizens. It is a cultural phenomenon peculiar to black Americans, and it is a posture so close to paranoid thinking that the mental disorder into which black people most frequently fall is paranoid psychosis...Can we say that white men have driven black men mad? (Grier and Cobbs, 1969, pp.172–73)[26]

In many ways, the chronic struggle to succeed and the strong potential for hostility among the Type-A individual is similar to the paradoxical problem that confronts many black people in the United States. They are born into a societal system where dark skin color and being black has historically been devalued and associated with a limited potential to produce positive consequences within the society. On the one hand, black American are encouraged to strive to succeed, to control their surroundings, and to adopt industrial virtues that reflect hard work, punctuality, perseverance, loyalty, and obedience. Black children and adolescents are told that they are the masters of their destiny.

But are blacks in the United States really in control of their destiny? Are black people trying to control the uncontrollable or reach the unreachable? I think that the answers to these questions are very complex and that many black Americans are trapped or stuck in a social-psychological situation where there is a willingness to entertain the notion of the American Dream. At the same time, however, there is a strong sense that they are powerless and that the struggle to achieve success will not be rewarded. There is a forever widening gap between blacks and whites in the social, economic, and health circumstances in the United States. Considering these realities, I wonder if there is any worthwhile purpose in encouraging young black Americans to do something that may not be possible.

At present, the unemployment rate among blacks is so miserable that it is difficult to estimate accurately. The drop-out rate for black children in many cities is extremely high, and a disproportionate number of black kids are tracked into slow-learning classes where they have no possible chance of obtaining an academic background that is suitable for gaining entry to college or the job market. If the primary basis for male (and female) identity in our society is the job you have and the work you do, then the inability of black men to gain meaningful employment means that they are nothing—people without an identity. Ultimately, this downward spiral results in a loss of self-respect and further economic crises for black families.

The situation among many blacks is that the tools to implement changes are hidden or attainable only by suppressing one's aggressive drives and feelings of anger in order to be perceived as attractive, popular, pleasing, and in demand as a consumer product in a mass public market. In my opinion, the push toward success can leave a bitter aftertaste because of the need to pull away from strong and supportive bonds with family that is created by the desire to be successful and obtain the rewards of industrial society. What happens is that you are criticized and devalued if you do not strive to be successful, but you are criticized and devalued if you do. In other words, it does not matter what you have done or accomplished, who you accomplished it with, or where you accomplished whatever: The simple truth is that if you are black you are at the bottom of the ladder—the last to be hired, the first to be fired.

In the not so distant past, the evidence of institutional racism radiated throughout the land. Blacks had no doubt that they were living in a racist society: Schools, housing, restaurants, restrooms, and water fountains were segregated. But today, black youth are encouraged to believe that the battle against racism and segregation are over and that they have equal rights to the resources of the society. When, inevitably, racism is encountered—and it has taken on some rather sophisticated and covert characteristics—anger, hostility, and rage are often the result. Yet blacks may be more likely than whites to suppress—rather than express—these strong emotions.

There is little doubt that being black in the United States is tough. Even among well-educated black people who have achieved a certain degree of success in their careers, it is an everyday experience to cope with unjust situations that can be linked to the color of their skin. Although officially neither segregation nor discrimination exist in today's society, racial prejudice persists. Well-to-do or upwardly mobile black Americans may protect themselves psychologically by identifying with the "old black culture,"but many young blacks think of themselves simply as Americans. Yet, while on the one hand they may have rejected their black group identity, on the other hand they are not totally accepted by the rest of the U. S. society.

Though many of today's well-educated black Americans' social values, language, and behavior are identical to those of other Americans, the young upwardly mobile black man or woman is racially tied to and grouped with the stereotypes of black culture. Whereas the rest of society thinks of U. S. born blacks who are well-to-do or upwardly mobile as blacks, many of the black people who struggle day-to-day to make ends meet think of these more mobile blacks as "oreos"—a most uncomplimentary term used to describe U. S. born blacks who identify with white Americans. Thus, the U. S. born blacks who are well-educated and upwardly mobile face rejection on both sides. Perhaps this loss of group identity and the double rejection explain partially why anger, hostility, and aggression are thought to be more prevalent among black Americans compared to whites.

No matter how much we want to believe that the situation for American blacks is alright, it is not! For example, regardless of income, education, or occupational achievements, most blacks do not live in integrated neighborhoods. Conversely, blacks are exposed to higher crime rates, less effective educational systems, higher mortality risks, more dilapidated surroundings, and a poorer socioeconomic environment than whites—simply because of the persistently strong barriers to residential integration. Mounting evidence suggests that a large segment of working-age black men (15–44 percent) are alcoholics or drug abusers, are in prisons, unemployed, infected with the AIDS virus, or suffering from some other life-threatening condition.[27,28] Hypertension, for example, is estimated to be ten times more likely as the cause of death in black men compared to white men under 45 years of age.[29,30] For the most part, black males are the most feared group in our society; and the negative stereotypes—lazy, unintelligent, untrainable, violent troublemaker, drug abuser, abandoner of family—continue to be reinforced by the major formal and informal institutions of our society. But are blacks angry about these perceived and felt social and economic injustices that are part of the day-to-day struggle? Is there a difference in the anger experience and expression (or lack of) for blacks and whites? Given the long-standing link between hypertension and suppressed anger, and the fact that hypertension affects a greater percentage of black Americans, it seems logical that the difference in hypertension prevalences for blacks and whites would be explained by differences in the experience and expression of anger.

Basically, the few available studies looking at anger in blacks suggest that the expression of angry and hostile feelings—rather than the frequent experience of anger—is a greater problem for blacks than for whites. The bulk of the evidence shows that blacks are less likely than whites to express feelings of anger openly. This pattern of coping with anger is consistent with the historical and social analyses presented by psychologist Kenneth Clark and the two psychiatrists William Grier and Price Cobb. Basically, these scholars have proposed that blacks are forced or trapped into social and psychological positions where they feel threatened, angry, and hostile—yet they must suppress the expression of these emotions. E. Baughman has also argued that, for the most part blacks tend to avoid dealing with anger—especially that provoked by whites—by resorting to behaviors such as: (1) displacement of aggression onto other blacks (a possible cause of the increased black-on-black crime and homicide rates); (2) attempts to remain unaffected by such feelings (denial, staying cool); (3) wit and humor; and (4) identification with the oppressor (whites).[32] No matter which of these responses you consider, none of them represents a full acknowledgment of the degree of the experience of anger or an open expression of the angry feelings. Therefore, it would appear that much of the anger in blacks is unresolved or repressed, and this could very well account for the perception among whites of the angry and hostile attitudes among blacks.

Research conducted in the 1970s and earlier revealed that blacks and whites differ in their tendencies toward anger, primarily suppressed anger. For example, Crain and Weisman found that blacks and many poorly educated individuals are much less likely to recall angry feelings experienced in the past than their white and/or highly educated black counterparts.[33] In an earlier study, Yarrow found that, when black children are faced with provocation, they tended to be more covert (fearful, anxious, withdrawn from others) in their expression of emotions—rather than engage in overt behaviors such as fighting and using obscene language.

In one of the most interesting studies conducted in the 1970s, psychologist W. Doyle Gentry observed that black males were more likely to suppress their expression of anger than black females when provoked in an experimental situation designed to be frustrating.[35] In other words, both male and female black college students reported increased anger, and had heightened blood pressure and verbal aggressiveness on being insulted by the white examiner, but only the black females overtly and openly expressed their dislike and disapproval of the person delivering the insult. Therefore, these findings suggest that, for blacks, gender is strongly related to the expression of anger.

In order to clarify the relationship between gender and anger expression for blacks, I used data from the National Survey of Black Americans (NSBA)—see Chapter 2—to determine if adult black males and females are different from each other in how they cope with disturbing life events. In other words, respondents were asked to rate how they act or feel emotionally during the occurrence of negative life events that make them think they are at the point of a nervous breakdown. Black women were more likely to report that they lost their temper and had fights and arguments with others during these times, compared to black males. Other results revealed that black women respond to these stressful times by being more depressed (feeling lonely, crying easily; having a poor appetite; not being able to get going) and anxious (feeling jumpy or jittery; sleeping restlessly) than black males. Black males, on the other hand, were more likely to report that they would drink alcohol or get high in other ways as a means of coping with stressful times that are so bad they are at the point of a nervous breakdown. In essence, the results for black men suggest that repression may be the chief means of coping with personal stress. In other words, black men deny feeling bad and depressed about their personal difficulties, but they engage in those self-destructive behaviors that often accompany the experience of psychologic distress.

With regard to anger being more outwardly expressed by black females during times of intense personal stress, this is similar to data I derived from audio-recordings of the responses of black male and female college students to questions about anger. Basically, the black females were more expressive, spoke in a louder tone of voice, and exhibited more signs of irritability during these interviews than their male counterparts. Interestingly enough, the blood pressure readings of black females were more reactive—achieved higher levels—than the males as they responded to questions about the relationship between anger and recent stress in their lives.

Perhaps the males in this study were attempting to maintain their cool and to appear as if they were not emotionally or physiologically affected by the interview. Males may also have been responding to the interview questions with answers that were more socially acceptable or that would be perceived as being masculine. In either case, with conflicts about the expression of anger being such a consistent characteristic among blacks, one cannot help but wonder if the expression of anger (or lack of) is related to other factors in the day-to-day lives of blacks. Interestingly enough, this question was one of the reasons for a study conducted by Jaculine Fleming.[36] In this study, the relationship between suppressed hostility and academic performance was examined within a sample of black college students. Although black students expressed their anger less frequently than white students, suppressed anger was strongly correlated with test scores on the Scholastic Aptitude Test (SAT) for black students attending New York University.

More recent evidence that blacks and whites tend toward different styles of coping with anger was revealed by W. Doyle Gentry.[37] Using data from a study of 1,006 adult residents of Detroit, Gentry and his associates showed that black and white adult Americans differ somewhat in their habitual propensity for expressing across a wide range of anger-provoking interpersonal situations. Overall, the findings showed that black males as well as individuals residing in high-stress neighborhoods are more likely to suppress their expression of anger.

As reviewed in Chapter 3, blood pressure and the percentage of individuals with hypertension was greater among those residents of Detroit who were more likely to suppress their expression of anger. Further work by Gentry and his associates showed that the suppressed anger-coping style mediates the relationship between elevated blood pressure and both job and family strain. Job strain referred to the failure to have: (1) a chance to earn more money, (2) a chance to work with friendly people, (3) the chance to learn new skills or use one's present skills, (4) a chance for job security, or (5) a chance to advance at work. Similarly, family strain referred to self-acknowledged failure to: (1) spend time with spouse, (2) make decisions with spouse, (3) have good sex with spouse, (4) receive appreciation from spouse, or (5) spend time with children and be a good parent. Basically, the analysis of these data revealed that blacks and whites who are high in either type of life strain and who also suppress anger in day-to-day life situations run the risk of significantly elevated blood pressure, compared to those individuals who have low levels of life strain and/or openly express their anger.

Some additional findings by Gentry and his associates show that the manner in which one copes with anger mediates the relationship between elevated blood pressure and interracial hostility. Individuals who were high in interracial hostility (i.e., responding positively to "Sometimes I hate white people," "When I'm in a place where all of the people are white, I often feel I'm in enemy territory," and "I am most at ease when I am with blacks and there are no whites present") and who were more likely to suppress their anger had higher blood pressures than those persons low in interracial hostility and/or those who openly express their feelings of anger when provoked. Interestingly enough, only 36 percent (172 persons) of the 480 black adults in this investigation had high levels of interracial hostility, and the majority of individuals with a high level of interracial hostility had normal blood pressures.

Taken together, the findings above indicate that black adults are more likely than whites to suppress and not openly express feelings of anger. Moreover, it has been speculated that anger suppression among black Americans may represent an overlearned self-control of anger that was adaptive early on in adjusting to the slave culture, yet persists to a certain degree today with some maladaptive consequences. Although many of the sources for the strong fear of counteraggression—fear of physical harm to self and family—that have inhibited blacks from openly expressing anger have been removed or outlawed in our society, several sources do remain (e.g., lack of economic empowerment) and are likely to be behind the lack of open expression of many emotions among black Americans for a long time to come. Nevertheless, in thinking about the origin of the suppressed-anger coping style, one must examine whether its existence among blacks is due solely to the fear of counteraggression from people with power, or whether it can be traced to family relationships during childhood?

Fortunately, W. Doyle Gentry and his associates addressed this very issue. Their data derived from the study of black and white adults in Detroit suggest that anger-coping styles are learned during childhood and appear to be related to parental disciplinary styles. For example, of individuals who admitted in retrospect that they had behaved in a rebellious manner by "resisting parental punishment" rather than acting submissive and "giving in," a greater percentage were persons classified as Anger-Out (79 percent) compared to Anger-In (21 percent). Both black and white respondents classified as Anger-In were more likely to remember their parents as loving, warm, close, easygoing, and relaxed individuals. In contrast, respondents classified as anger-out described their parents as being cold, strict,and tense.

Although this is a bit speculative, the pattern of these findings suggests that the chronic suppression of anger in adulthood may be as much a function of the individual's attempt to maintain the love connection as it is a function of the fear of counterattack. In other words, the catalyst behind the suppression of intense feelings of anger may be deeply rooted in the individual's need to be loved, fear of losing love, fear of being abandoned, or fear of upsetting the parents. Interesting in this regard are the findings from one of our studies of stressful life events in children—which shows that witnessing arguments between parents is one of the most distressing events for a child.[13]

In the Detroit Study, the outward expression of anger was presumably associated with a higher level of interpersonal problems between the parents and the child. The child who exhibited the Anger-In coping style may have been just as problematic as the Anger-Out child. However, the easygoing and relaxed disciplinary style of the parents of the Anger-In child may have contributed to the child's not being comfortable expressing anger—or any emotions for that matter. Perhaps, some black children who grow up in close, easygoing, and relaxed families are conditioned from an early age to pout and sulk and withdraw from people as a means of coping with angry feelings. In the context of the presence of stressful life events (e.g., witnessing parents argue; impoverishment due to low income and education level of parents), the child who suppresses rather than expresses anger may be more desirable and less of a problem for some parents. In this sense, it may be that submissiveness is one of the characteristics of individuals who chronically suppress anger as a means of coping with stressful provocations.

This is precisely one of the research issues that was addressed in three separate studies conducted by Dr. Stevo Julius at the University of Michigan.[38] In each of these studies, the patients with borderline hypertension were characterized as overly submissive and sociable according to the Cattell 16 Personality Factor questionnaire. How generalizable are these findings? One of the studies was completed in Yugoslavia—a country ethnically, socially, and economically quite different from the United States. Although the average scores for Yugoslavian subjects were somewhat different from U. S. subjects, borderline hypertensive patients were more submissive and sociable than normotensive control subjects. Even more directly in line with the notion that submissiveness is a characteristic of individuals who habitually suppress anger are the 1977 findings by Murray Esler that show borderline hypertensive subjects to be characterized by submissiveness and strong feelings of anger that are suppressed.[39] Finally, the results of one of my recent studies shows that young black men who are at risk for hypertension because their parents have hypertension are more submissive than black men without a parental history of hypertension.[40]

The men at risk also experience feelings of anger more frequently, and they have a more exaggerated cardiovascular response to stress than sons of normotensive parents. Taken together, these results suggest that the tendency to be submissive when provoked and the hyperreactive cardiovascular response to stressful events are possibly inherited.

With the exception of the research conducted by psychologist W. Doyle Gentry and his associates, very few studies have been conducted to examine differences in anger among blacks and whites. The research that I have conducted is based primarily on adolescents and young-adult college student volunteers.[6,7,40] Much like the rationale behind the study of adults in the Detroit Study, the purpose of my research on anger in black and white adolescents was to see if differences between blacks and whites in anger-coping styles would explain black–white differences in blood pressure. Well, as discussed in Chapter 3, the relationship between elevated blood pressure and measures of the expression and experience of anger is similar for black and white adolescents. Nevertheless, blacks and whites do differ from each other with regard to both the experience and the expression of anger.

In my research, black adolescent males and females do not differ from their white counterparts in their disposition to experience feelings of anger frequently. However, black females are likely to react with more intense feelings of anger than white females when evaluated unfairly or criticized. Most importantly, black adolescents of both sexes are more likely than their white peers to hold in and suppress feelings of anger. For example, black adolescents were as likely to report that they would get angry and keep their feelings to themselves when prevented from joining a club, or when a teacher got mad at them for something that wasn't their fault, and when someone cut in front of them at the movie and received the last ticket to the show. Regardless of the social context of the provocation, black adolescents are more likely than whites to suppress the expression of their anger. Furthermore, black adolescent males—but not the females—were more likely to report that they would feel guilty and sorry if they got angry or mad and expressed their anger in situations. Perhaps this is related to differences in disciplinary styles for blacks and whites, or these differences could be related to the degree that anger is openly expressed in black and white families.[41,42]

Another important issue relates to whether the suppressed-anger coping style is a consequence of the differential treatment that black youth (particularly males) receive at school for misbehaving. For example, it has been my observation that black students are disproportionately referred to the principal's office for punishment after having committed the same offenses as their white counterparts. There is also a tendency for both black and white teachers to blame the black student for arguments and fights with white students. On the one hand, it seems that we are telling black kids about the importance of education and academic competitiveness and aggressiveness; but on the other hand, we

consider the outward display of aggression to be deviant and delin-
quent. However, the questions and issues raised by this discussion must
await future research studies.

In the Spring of 1989 I conducted a survey in a group of black and
white adults.   Information about anger was obtained during a brief
interview; all participants had professional occupations (psychologist,
physician, psychotherapist, college counselor, medical technician) and
were between 22 and 46 years of age. The interview elicited information
about perceived differences in anger for blacks and whites in the five
areas summarized below.

1.   Causes of Anger—The question read, "Do you think that the
       causes for anger are different for blacks and whites in this country?"
       The results showed that 65 percent of the blacks and 50 percent of
       the whites thought that the causes for anger episodes are different
       for blacks and whites. More blacks than whites said they are likely to
       get angry where there is a violation of their rights or when they are
       treated unfairly and when racism is a part of the provocation.

2.   Reactions during anger episodes—Seventy percent of the blacks
       and 58 percent of the whites thought that blacks and whites differ
       in their reactions during anger. Although both blacks and whites
       thought that blacks are more likely to keep feelings of anger to
       themselves, a greater proportion of the blacks thought that the
       expression of anger (or lack of) would depend on the authority or
       rank of the person(s) involved in the provocation: Blacks would be
       more likely to suppress feelings if the person has a higher author-
       ity. The majority of blacks and whites (62 percent) thought that
       that blacks would be more likely to "take their anger out" on other
       blacks.

3.   Aftereffects of Anger—Sixty-five percent of the blacks thought that
       blacks and whites are not different in the kind of emotional reac-
       tions (guilt, shame, embarrassment, sadness) they feel following
       anger e pisodes, while 63 percent of the whites believed this to be
       true. Overall, both blacks and whites thought that blacks have
       more to lose than whites if anger is expressed in the work place and
       other public situations. On the other hand, the majority of blacks
       and whites thought that there would be no differences between
       blacks and whites in the degree of guilt, shame, embarrassment,
       and sadness experienced after anger episodes.

4.   Frequency of Anger Experiences—Basically, a slightly larger per-
       centage of blacks (60 percent) than whites (55 percent) thought
       that the frequency of anger episodes would be different for blacks
       and whites. Both blacks and whites thought that blacks would
       experience episodes more frequently than whites. The chief

reason given for this was that the day-to-day experiences of blacks are more likely to involve struggles in overcoming economic, racist, and stressful social circumstances where there is little chance for success.

5.   Crying—Eighty-five percent of the blacks thought that blacks and whites are similar when it comes to crying during and after an anger episode, while 75 percent of the whites also thought this to be true.

So there are differences between blacks and whites with regard to anger; but the differences have to do with the lack of expression of anger, and the circumstances that are the cause of the provocations. Overall, blacks appear to be no different than whites in their general disposition to experience anger frequently. Blacks—particularly females—are more likely to react with intense feelings of anger when confronted with stressful social situations that involve criticisms and unfair evaluations. Both black males and females are also more likely to suppress the expression of anger when provoked. Basically, I think that these differences are related to the manner in which parents model anger coping behaviors—which in turn is probably related to differences in parental disciplinary styles among blacks, relative to whites. It is also my belief that our educational system is partly to blame for the low level of assertiveness and diminished expression of emotions among blacks. Furthermore, as between men and women, there may also be differences in the rules of conversation for blacks and whites—which could contribute to the dominant-culture stereotype that anger is more of a problem for blacks.

ANGER DOWN UNDER

But what about differences in anger between cultures? Unfortunately, the idea that anger can be reliably and validly measured is still new to many psychologists. However, a method of generating and experiencing a sequence of emotions—anger, hate, grief, love, sex, joy, reverence—referred to as "Sentic Cycles," has been investigated by Manfred Clynes at the University of Melbourne in Australia.[43] With this method, the subjects are encouraged to generate a series of emotions, usually from recall of the feelings, thoughts, and bodily sensations associated with the emotions. Each emotion is then rated according to its intensity on a scale of 0 through 5 (0 = no effect, 5 = maximal intensity). Clynes's data were obtained from a sample of more than 1,000 subjects collected over a ten-year period. Subjects were U. S. and Australian adults from 18 to 76 years old.

A comparison of females and males in the U.S. and Australian samples revealed that, of the seven emotions, love achieved the highest intensity rating; next came joy; then sex and grief, anger, reverence and hate the lowest. Overall, U.S. men and U.S. women were very similar in the intensity of most emotions, but the men rated anger and hate more intensely than the women did. These differences indicate a somewhat greater open aggressiveness among men than women in the United States. In this study, Australian women scored strikingly similar to U.S. women on most emotions, except that they scored substantially lower for hate and somewhat higher for grief than U.S. women. Perhaps this difference is partly related to differences in the sociologic conditions of the two countries. For example, Australian women are not so emancipated and independent as U. S. women. The higher ratings of grief among Australian women—probably because grief has not turned into hate as it often may have for U.S. women—is consistent with the view that there is a greater acceptance of repression among Australian women. Australian men scored significantly lower than Australian women on all emotions except sex, and lower than U. S. men on all emotions. As remarkable as these results may appear, they reflect Australian mores and an educational system that teaches it is unmanly to show emotion, except at sporting events.

7

Regulating Anger and Other Exaggerated Emotional Responses to Stress

As the discussions throughout this book attest, research on the role of the AHA! Syndrome in physical and emotional disorders is progressing at a steady rate. At the present time, anger, hostility, and aggression are seriously implicated in the etiology and maintenance of essential hypertension, coronary heart disease, and cancer. Also, there is some convincing evidence that elements of the AHA! Syndrome are related to classic risk factors such as total cholesterol, alcohol intake, and cigarette smoking. The inappropriate management and expression of anger and hostility are central elements involved in both child abuse and spouse abuse. Sufficient evidence also exists to indicate that the experience of anger is amplified by alcohol intake, and by talking about anger episodes—both of which strongly influence cognitive appraisal of the provocation.

While research on the relationship between the AHA! Syndrome and health is progressing, the behavioral and psychological treatment of anger, hostility, and aggression[1,2] has lagged far behind the systematic treatment of chronic problems with anxiety and depression.[3] The major reasons for the lack of research on the management of anger are discussed in various manuscripts by psychologist Raymond Novaco.[4-6] First of all, measurement of the experience, expression, and control of anger is more difficult than the measurement of other emotions such as anxiety or depression. For example, in the case of anxiety, there are a number of systematic and validated procedures for inducing anxiety: presenting the subject with difficult tasks; providing negative performance evaluations. Second, unlike anxiety and depression where there are several clinical diagnostic categories, there are no formal diagnostic criteria for the AHA! Syndrome. Other unique problems that have been identified as hindering the systematic treatment of anger include these observations: (1) therapists and counselors are often uneasy about working with persons who have anger management problems; (2) poor treatment outcome is associated with working with persons who have explosive tempers (e.g., prisoners, juvenile delinquents, child and spouse abusers); and (3) proneness to anger and aggression can often frustrate individuals who are impatient about vague and ambiguous treatment goals.

Although there are a number of problems associated with the psychotherapeutic treatment of anger–aggression problems, the harmful effects of the AHA! Syndrome on psychological well-being and health argue for the development of psychologically–based interventions. In this regard, the purpose of this chapter is to review the psychological treatment and intervention approaches that have been developed to help individuals manage and modify anger, hostility, and aggression. Rather than provide an exhaustive review of the research in this area, I will outline various therapeutic intervention strategies and provide references where more information can be found. The second section of this chapter contains a brief review of stress and anger–hostility management in the treatment of hypertension and Type-A behavior, and the final section describes some general strategies for managing stress and irritability.

THERAPEUTIC INTERVENTION STRATEGIES

A number of procedures for the management of Anger–Hostility–Aggression problems have been reported in the psychological literature over the past 30 years. Nevertheless, the psychotherapeutic interventions that have received research evaluations basically fall into one of four groups: (1) behavioral therapy using a procedure known as "systematic desensitization"; (2) behavioral interventions using operant conditioning therapies; (3) training in assertiveness and social skills; and (4) cognitive-behavioral treatment approaches.

Systematic Desensitization

The systematic desensitization to anger typically involves: (1) training in deep muscle relaxation to compete with feelings of physical arousal, anxiety, and irritation; (2) construction of a hierarchy of situations ranked by the individual from least to most anger provoking; and (3) counterpoising relaxation while the person imagines that the actual hierarchy situation is taking place. Basically, the individual is instructed to imagine each of the hierarchy situations from least anger provoking to most anger provoking, while remaining in a relaxed and calm manner.

The process responsible for systematic desensitization—as presented by Dr. Joseph Wolpe, who developed this technique—is called "reciprocal inhibition."[7] It is assumed that, if a response inhibitory to anger can be made to occur in the presence of the anger-provoking situation so that it is accompanied by a complete or partial suppression of the anger response, the bond or link between the anger-provoking situation and the anger response will be weakened.[8]

Thus, a young man who gets extremely angry when his work performance is critically evaluated by his supervisor could be taught relaxation and breathing exercises prior to meeting with the supervisor. The therapist generally helps him to pinpoint the situations that cause him to feel angry and hostile. For example, thinking about all of the hard work and long hours that went into the project, setting a time to meet with the supervisor, listening to the supervisor's criticisms are ranked in increasing order of their anger-hostility provoking capacity for the man. The man is then taught how to relax and to imagine each of these events while remaining calm and relaxed.

In one study in this area, R. E. Smith used humor as the incompatible response conditioned to the anger-provoking situations.[9] Basically, the deep muscle relaxation training proved to be ineffective for a particular client, and—rather than abandon the case—Smith had the woman develop a "humor hierarchy" that enabled her to view the anger situations from a new perspective and develop coping responses incompatible with being angry.

Operant Conditioning Therapies

Under the operant conditioning procedures based on the laboratory investigations of B. F. Skinner, it is more important to explore the effect or consequences of behavior than to know what caused the behavior in the first place.[10] Behaviors that are modified or maintained by the consequences that follow them are called "operants". Operant behaviors are so called because they operate on or influence the environment, which results in additional consequences that strengthen or weaken the behavior. In other words, operants constitute what persons do or say as they interact with the environment, and the consequences of these behaviors are often either pleasant or aversive for the individual. In operant conditioning, positive or pleasant consequences (positive reinforcement) are used to increase the frequency of desired behavior, while negative or aversive consequences (negative reinforcement) are generally used to decrease the frequency of undesirable behaviors.

Psychologist G. R. Patterson and his colleagues at the Oregon Social Learning Center are foremost in using operant conditioning therapies to treat anger–hostility management problems.[11–14] Their intervention program has been extremely successful in teaching parents how to use social and consumable reinforcers to increase desirable behaviors, and negative reinforcements to reduce coercive temper tantrums and annoying reactions of angry and aggressive children. The intervention program at Oregon, for the most part, has shown that reductions in angry and aggressive behavior of a target child is associated with an overall reduction in the level of coerciveness and anger for all family members.

Assertiveness and Social Skills

One therapeutic approach to anger assumes that problems concerning management of anger, hostility, and aggression are the result of the individual's having a deficit in social skills. Because of this deficit, the individual often responds to situations involving interpersonal conflict, stress, or disputes with intense feelings of anger and hostility. This often leads to avoidance, threats, antagonistic thoughts, and other hostile behaviors, minimizing the chances that anger will be used as a signal of something wrong and that the problem will be dealt with and resolved. The assertiveness and social-skills approach to the treatment of anger-hostility involves teaching the individual how to utilize appropriate alternatives to manage anger effectively, thereby altering the probability that it will escalate to hostility and aggressive behaviors.[15-17]

Although there are a number of treatment strategies that fall into the category of assertiveness and social-skills training, the results from these approaches are mixed. Training in assertiveness and social skills often includes: (1) modeling of appropriate behavioral alternatives; (2) having the individual engage in role-play and rehearse the behavioral responses that are chosen to be the alternative to hostile and aggressive reactions; and (3) pinpointing problem behaviors so that feedback and reinforcement of the alternative responses is consistent. As indicated earlier, these treatment approaches have not always been effective with regard to modifying abusive verbal outbursts or reducing fights and arguments among distressed couples or families with children who have conduct problems.

Cognitive-Behavioral Techniques

The area in which the majority of intervention programs have been focused is the cognitive-behavioral treatment approach to the management of negative emotional states which is rooted in the early clinical work of Aaron Beck[3] and Albert Ellis.[1,2] Application of their findings to the management of anger started with the research of psychologist Raymond Novaco.[4-6]

The basic model of anger-related behavioral problems assumes that anger becomes a problem when it occurs too frequently, intensely, or long and when it leads to hostility and aggression. Other anger-related behavioral problems include a disruption in relationships at work and within one's family, and the occurrence of physical problems such as chest pains, hypertension, and gastric distress. Anger is viewed as being the result of both external and internal factors. External factors might include frustrations, annoying and irritating situations, verbal and physical abuse, unfair treatment, and critical evaluations of one's performance or character. Internal factors such as thoughts, expectations, and self-statements (the things we tell ourselves) are thought to influence our affective state, bodily responses (muscle tension, in particular), tolerance for dealing with provocations, and the degree of ill-humor (taking things too seriously; being moody, cross, and sour) associated with the provocation. Moreover, two basic courses of action or styles of behaving are thought to contribute to anger. The first is withdrawal–avoidance (Anger–In). Although the person continues to think about the situations that are the source of anger, he or she ultimately becomes discouraged and loses all sense of self-worth. Such a person may become depressed and direct anger inward, which could increase the sensitivity to unpleasant events and feelings of depression and helplessness. The second course of action is antagonism–hostility–aggression (Anger-Out). In this style of behavior, feelings of anger and irritability often escalate to hostility and aggressive behaviors that are openly expressed at people and objects in the environment.

The cognitive-behavioral intervention technique is designed to promote adaptive coping with provocations, and it emphasizes cognitive mediation and reciprocal relationships between external environmental and internal cognitive, emotional, and physiological processes. The treatment procedures are therefore based on the conviction that emotional arousal and the cause of action that such arousal instigates are defined or determined by one's cognitive structuring of the provocation situation.

The core components of the cognitive-behavioral intervention program consists of: (1) teaching the individual in cognitive mediation techniques (how to assess anger; cognitive restructuring; problem-solving skills, self-instruction); and (2) arousal and emotional reduction methods (primarily, deep muscle relaxation). Thus, a person with a problem managing anger-hostility-aggression would undergo initial treatment sessions that focused on cognitive preparation. The person would be introduced to the rationale of the treatment approach, and then asked to keep a diary of the frequency, intensity, and duration of anger episodes and to identify situations that trigger anger. During the skills acquisition phase at the second or third session, the person is taught relaxation skills and encouraged to maintain a sense of humor as a response to anger—not to take things too seriously. The person is taught how to dissect a provocation experience into a sequence of stages that consist of: (1) preparation for the provocation; (2) dealing with the confrontation and its impact; (3) coping with physiologic and emotional arousal; and (4) coping with subsequent reflections about the provocation by altering self-statement about the event. The individual is encouraged to role-play and practice using the cognitive-behavioral intervention techniques by exposing him or her to regulated doses of the anger-provoking circumstances. It has been demonstrated that these activities help facilitate learning how to cope effectively with aroused angry feelings and teach the person how to distinguish anger from hostility and aggression.[4,5]

The cognitive-behavioral program for managing anger has been systematically used in a number of studies. For example, Novaco first used this technique as a treatment for hospitalized patients with severe anger problems,[5] and with occupational groups such as police officers who are at high risk both for being the recipient of angry outbursts and for reacting to stressful situations with anger.[6] In one study, probation officers who were trained to administer this form of therapy became more proficient in helping their clients deal with anger. Psychologists Joseph Denicola and Jack Sandler used a variation of the cognitive-behavioral treatment strategies and obtained decreases in anger and aggressive behaviors in both parents and children undergoing a program for abusive parents.[18] Feindler and Fremouw used the procedure in the treatment of adolescents with anger problems.[19]

STRESS MANAGEMENT IN THE TREATMENT OF HYPERTENSION AND TYPE-A BEHAVIOR

As you know by now, hypertension is one of the most important public health problems facing the United States today. It is estimated that approximately 60 million adult Americans are at increased health risk due to elevated blood pressure. A recognizable specific cause—such as kidney disease or narrowing of the renal arteries—is found in only 15 percent of patients with hypertension, while the blood pressure problem cannot be attributed to any known organic cause in 85 percent of hypertension patients.[20,21] It is generally acknowledged that blood pressure is determined by many factors (e.g., age, gender, diet, family history or genetic factors) and that the psychosocial and physical environment (e.g., noisy and stressful living conditions) may play some role in the development of hypertension for some individuals.

In view of this acceptance of the multifactorial nature of hypertension, the prescribing of pharmacologic agents should no be regarded as only one of several approaches to the treatment of hypertension. In considering the stress-management or arousal-reduction strategies for treating hypertension, one must differentiate among a number of approaches—including progressive muscle relaxation, autogenic relaxation training, biofeedback, meditation, and combinations of these techniques.[22,23] These nonpharmacologic therapies have been particularly recommended for individuals with mild forms of hypertension. Another reason for these therapies is an outgrowth of concerns about pharmacotherapy, including adverse side effects, potential negative consequences of antihypertensive medications, patient noncompliance with pharmacologic regimen—which can be as high as 70 percent—and the high cost of medication. There is also a growing concern that antihypertensive medications raise certain lipoprotein and cholesterol levels, and some medications have been associated with an unusually high rate of mortality for individuals with electrocardiographic abnormalities.

The need to develop nonpharmacologic therapies is strengthened by the fact that these approaches have particular relevance for patients with mild hypertension: 70 percent of U.S. hypertensives are considered to have mild hypertension. Although these techniques do not typically produce large reductions in blood pressure—5–10 mmHg—they have demonstrated consistent and reliable decreases. Moreover, the Hypertension Detection and Follow-up Program has demonstrated that a reduction in diastolic blood pressure of approximately 5mmHg is sufficient to result in an approximately 17-percent reduction in the mortality rate over a 5-year period.[24] In fact, the greatest benefit is noted in the mild hypertensive category, with a 4.3 mmHg reduction in diastolic blood pressure accounting for a 20-percent or more reduction in the mortality rate. Because of the overall significance of these results, the 1984 U.S. Joint National Committee on Detection, Evaluation, and Treatment of Blood Pressure recommended stress-management or arousal-reduction therapies in the context of a comprehensive hypertension treatment program.[25]

Although there are literally hundreds of studies on stress management approaches to the treatment of hypertension,[26-28] the most recent reviews of these studies have found average reductions of 10 mmHg (systolic blood pressure) and 7 mmHg (diastolic blood pressure) for the arousal-reduction and relaxation therapies. Furthermore, Dr. Chandra Patel has successfully used combinations of relaxation and pharmacologic therapies both to lower blood pressure and to reduce or eliminate dependence on medication for a significant proportion of the patients enrolled in her studies.[29–33] In fact, Patel and her associates conducted the most comprehensive series of studies of arousal-reduction therapies to date. The most recent study in this series demonstrated maintenance of significant reductions in blood pressure over a 4-year period in patients with hypertension. In addition to demonstrating that arousal-reduction therapies are effective in the treatment of hypertensive patients, Dr. Patel's work has provided unique evidence that stress management can prevent hypertension among individuals with normal blood pressure but who have other risk factors for coronary heart disease -- high serum cholesterol and cigarette smoking. Basically, the 4-year follow-up of these patients revealed that blood pressure and other CHD risk factors were significantly lower when compared with a control group that did not receive the stress management treatment.[32] Overall, these findings clearly indicate that patients with identifiable risk factors for CHD can achieve preventive benefits from stress management and relaxation training.

One of the most recent and interesting studies of the nonpharmacologic management of hypertension was reported in 1989 by Judith Achmon, Michel Granek, Mira Golomb, and Jacob Hart.[34] In this study, the effects of two psychological treatments for essential hypertension were compared. Hypertensive patients were randomly assigned to either: (1) cognitive therapy for anger control; (2) biofeedback for heart-rate control; or (3) a no-treatment control group. Results of the Achmon study will be discussed further on. The two treatments it chose to investigate are of interest here in themselves, however. Anger-control cognitive therapy aims to reduce the level of anger and to change its overt expression so that fewer life situations that trigger anger arousal will be perceived as anger provoking. The rationale for heart-rate biofeedback has to do with the notion that one cause of essential hypertension is an elevated cardiac output and elevated heart rate. Furthermore, elevated heart rate in youth—independent of blood pressure level—is a predictor of hypertension later in life.[35-37] Several studies have shown that hypertensive patients are able to control their blood pressure through biofeedback and that training subjects to modify their heart rate is associated with a simultaneous change in blood pressure.[38,39] In the usual sense, heart-rate biofeedback is a procedure used to teach an individual how voluntarily to lower the heart-rate response to laboratory events. This is usually accomplished by monitoring the heart rate and other physiological variables while the subject learns to control his or her heart rate. As a result of controlling and lowering the heart-rate response, there is a lower blood-pressure response to events in the laboratory and a generalized calmer response to life situations outside of the laboratory.

As indicated above, the study by Achmon and colleagues was quite impressive.[34] Basically, its main results were that: (1) both psychological treatment methods resulted in a significant decrease in blood pressure as compared with the no-treatment control group; (2) the decrease in blood pressure was greater for the heart-rate biofeedback group, and (3) a greater reduction and control of anger was achieved with cognitive therapy. Further, the findings show that, after six months of follow-up, the average blood pressure for both psychological treatment methods remained significantly lower than before therapy. Whereas psychological approaches to the management of essential hypertension have been criticized for being beneficial to only a small number of patients, approximately 40 and 54 percent—respectively—of the patients assigned to cognitive and biofeedback therapy achieved a decrease in blood that was sufficient to normalize their blood pressure.

In a related study, the effects of relaxation therapy on blood pressure and the neurohumoral response to anger provocation was studied in a group of 30 male patients with mild hypertension.[40] Of these patients, 13 did not receive training in relaxation—the No=Relax Group. The seventeen other patients were taught a progressive muscle-relaxation exercise—the Relax Group. Prior to therapy, the anger-provocation procedures induced increases in systolic and diastolic blood pressure in both the No-Relax (143/91 increased to 155/96) and Relax (139/88 increased to 146/91) groups, and plasma norepinephrine was increased from 280 to 307 pg/ml for all patients. After therapy, there was a 30 percent increase in norepinephrine (213 increased to 277 pgml) during anger provocation for the No-Relax Group and no significant change in the Relax group (226 increased to 235 pgml). Relaxation therapy also reduced the resting level of diastolic blood pressure and the systolic response to anger provocation was significantly lower.

As indicated at the beginning of this chapter, research on the psychological treatment of Anger–Hostility–Aggression has lagged far behind the research demonstrating relationships between the AHA! Syndrome and health problems. Thus, one can only speculate about the possible long term impact and effectiveness of combining an anger management program with pharmacologic therapies to treat hypertension. Given the link between anger-hostility and elevated blood pressure, it is surprising that to date there are so few systematic studies of the management of the AHA! Syndrome in hypertensive patients. On the other hand, a number of recent studies have used combinations of anxiety and anger management training to alter Type-A behavior.[41–49] For example, Ethel Roskies has developed a systematic program that is the result of ten years of testing with healthy Type-A managers and professionals.[45,49] The basic premise of her program is that there is no way to identify in advance all the situations in which an exaggerated response or hyperreactivity to stress is likely to occur, nor all the forms that it is likely to take. Instead, to effect real and lasting change in the habitual management of stress, the individual is taught how to function independently and to devise and implement coping strategies that alter bad and unpleasant stress perceptions and events.

For the most part, the various stress and anger–anxiety management programs are successful in reducing Type-A behavior, and these results are often corroborated by reports from spouses, co-workers, and friends. The most striking evidence in support of the importance of stress management and arousal-reduction therapies in altering Type-A behavior was reported by Meyer Friedman and associates as part of the Recurrent Coronary Prevention Project.[46–48] In this study, 862 patients who had suffered a myocardial infarction volunteered to be randomly selected and enrolled into: (1) an experimental section of 592 patients, who received a standard group cardiologic counseling in addition to Type-A behavioral counseling; and (2) a control group of 270 patients, who received only the cardiologic counseling.

The Type-A counseling consisted of training in progressive muscle relaxation, recognition of causes and modification of exaggerated emotional reactions to stress, and other self-observational and self-assessment techniques.   This study is important because it demonstrated a reduction in Type-A behavior at the end of three years in 43.8 percent of the 592 participants who were enrolled in the sessions that received Type-A behavioral counseling in addition to group cardiologic counseling. More importantly, the three-year cumulative cardiac recurrence rate was 7.2 percent among participants who received the Type-A behavioral counseling and group cardiologic counseling, in comparison to 13 percent for those participants who were initially enrolled to receive only cardiologic counseling. The overall outcome of this study suggests that Type-A behavior can be altered in postinfarction patients and that such alteration is associated with a significantly reduced rate of nonfatal myocardial infarctions. Given the multidimensional nature of the Type-A behavioral counseling program, it is difficult to determine exactly whether each of the components of the therapy contributed to the subsequent reduction in myocardial infarctions. Perhaps the management of Anger—Hostility–Aggression is the only treatment component responsible for the reduction ? Future research may shed some light on this question.

GENERAL STRATEGIES FOR MANAGING ANGER AND IRRITABILITY

Anger and stressful situations can not be avoided, but they can be diffused. For some of us it takes a long time to diffuse the tension, anxieties, and feelings of irritability, while others can bring forth a speedy resolution to the provocation. Each of us is different; we have our own views of what might be the best technique for managing anger and stress. The techniques discussed in this section are quite simple and natural. Although I can not take credit for developing the techniques, I can assure you that I have personally found them useful in managing the tensions and feelings of irritability in my life.

Mellow Sounds

Although the research in this area is a bit new, it has been theorized that high-intensity sounds—noise—can alter physiological processes such as functioning of the cardiovascular, endocrine, respiratory, and digestive systems.[50–52] Therefore, playing soothing music can help individuals to relax and cope with stressful events (e.g., minor surgery, dental work). What convinced me of this was to listen to hard rock and roll and then soothing classical music without lyrics while my blood pressure was being measured over a 24-hour period. My heart rate and blood pressure were substantially lower during the soothing classical music. While I was listening to rock and roll, however, my blood pressure rose 15–30 mmHg higher than my resting levels.

In my experiences I have found it best to select relaxation music that is a bit slow, very quiet, and without lyrics. Such music has a pleasurable effect on my body, mind, and emotions. To a certain extent, my threshold for dealing with stress and anger-provoking events is noticeably elevated after mellowing out with soft sounds. In other words, I am not so likely to become impatient and irritated by the many everyday situations that would usually make my blood boil. So the next time you find yourself stuck in traffic, tune the radio to some mellow sounds. By the way, some people have discovered that singing and humming—while stuck in rush-hour traffic, for example—is an effective technique to calm the nerves and relax. I have also observed that I tend to sing and hum a bit more aggressively when I do the laundry—a tasks that I have not mastered.

Soaking Your Worries Away

For many of us the typical day begins and ends with a quick shower. In somewhere between 30 seconds and two minutes, we wash and clean our bodies. Who would deny just how great a hot shower feels after a long and hard day at the office or after engaging in strenuous yard word or exercise? Well, if it feels that great, why not get off your feet and stretch out in the tub and fully relax? Your answer to this question probably has something to do with our tendency to be always on the go and never have time for life's simple little pleasures.

Hot baths are great. Warm water causes the circulation to increase and calms you by relaxing muscles. I have found it useful and quite refreshing to enhance the tranquilizing effect of the bath by combining a warm bath with a progressive muscle relaxation exercise. These exercises are designed to enable the participant to tense and then relax each of the major muscle groups throughout the body. For example, while soaking up those suds, you can simply start by tensing your arms and keeping them tense until you count to ten, and then relaxing the arms. To complete the progressive muscle relaxation exercise, you will need to continue alternating between tensing and relaxing each of the major muscle groups throughout the body (face, neck, shoulders, back, buttock, thigh, legs). You can enhance the relaxation effect by listening to quiet music. What else can I say except—enjoy!

Physical Fitness and Emotionality

Regular physical activity has been shown to be an important variable in the maintenance and improvement of physical health and psychological well-being. Moreover, regular exercise is associated with such activities as reduced cardiovascular morbidity and mortality, normalization of carbohydrates and fat metabolism, lowering of blood pressure, and maintenance of ideal body weight.[53-55] Research concerning the role of exercise on psychological well-being, depression, and stress has revealed a high correlation between feeling good about your self and physical fitness. In other words, it has been demonstrated that an active exercise program reduces feelings of depression, anxiety, tension, and hostility.[56-58] Other psychological benefits of physical activity include improved self-image and feelings of confidence, and enhanced mental performance and concentration . In the case of walking, the most common form of exercise—it probably does not matter where you walk (e.g., through a scenic park, in a shopping mall, on a treadmill in a bare room) in order to gain the physical and emotional benefits of the activity. However, shuffling along with your eyes and head downward (the posture often associated with depression)—rather than walking in your regular stride—may be associated with negative emotions.

One study examined the effects of exercise on a laboratory rat in a cage placed inside another cage that held a hungry cat.[59] The situation was set up so that the cat could not physically get at the rat. One group of rats had an opportunity to engage in regular daily exercise on a running wheel that was placed within their cage, while a second group was denied access to the running wheel. The presence of the hungry cat was kept constant, however, and served as an extremely stressful daily event. When the rats were examined at the end of the study, the degree of cancerous tumor formation and abnormalities of the cardiovascular system were substantially higher for the rats that had been denied an opportunity to exercise on the running wheel. In other words, the results indicate that regular exercise buffers or minimizes the effects of stress on health.

In my own attempts to walk off tension and feelings of irritability, I have found it useful to promise myself that I will do my best not to think about whatever made me angry until I have finished my walk or jog. Interestingly enough, on one of those days when I was extremely upset about the status of a research project, I decided to go for a long jog at the end of the day. As usual I promised myself that I would not think about the situation until after my workout. As I was running through one of the most remote parts of the heavily wooded park, I came upon another jogger. It was obvious that we had startled each other and that both of us were using the jog to work off tension and negative feelings. I take pride in the fact that at that moment my complaints about my stressful day were being kept to myself. This is more than I can say for the other jogger, who was saying something like "damn, damn, damn——damn" as we ran past each other.

Appendixes

APPENDIX A: THE ELEMENTS OF ANGER AND SITUATIONAL
DETERMINANTS OF ANGER

Describe the situation that made you feel so angry that you thought you
were about at the point of—losing it, falling apart, a nervous breakdown:

_____

_____

_____

_____

_____

How intense was your anger?

1. Mild

2. Moderate

3. Severe

Was the cause of your anger?

1). Another person—Who?

_____

2). Yourself—Why?

_____

3). Some object (car, computer, etc.)

_____

Did your range of emotions include feeling:

	<u>No</u>	<u>Mild</u>	<u>Moderate</u>	<u>Severe</u>
1). Anxiety	1	2	3	4
2). Sadness	1	2	3	4
3). Depression	1	2	3	4
4). Hatred	1	2	3	4
5). Guilt	1	2	3	4
6). Happy	1	2	3	4
7). Fear	1	2	3	4

How long did you remain angry?

1. A few minutes

2. About an hour

3. An hour or more

4. Few hours

5. Half a day to a day

6. Few days

7. Week or more

How did you cope with the situation? _____

_____

What were the consequences of your actions and behavior?

_____

Did your actions make you feel?

1. Better

2. Worse

3. No Change

How did you express your feelings of anger?

1. Kept feelings to self

2. Showed your anger and expressed it

3. Remained calm and acted to solve the problem later

4. Immediately tried to solve the problem while staying calm

Test Yourself: Are there situations where you are more prone to anger?

Directions: A number of common social situations are given below. Read each situation and then circle (or simply note in your mind) the answer that best indicates the degree or amount of anger you would feel in the situation. There are no right or wrong answers. Do not spend too much time on any one situation, but give the answer that best describes the degree or amount of anger you would feel in the situation.

	Not At All Angry	Some- what Angry	Mode- rately Angry	Very Angry
1. You and your spouse (partner or significant other) have disagreements about social activities	1	2	3	4
2. You are criticized in front				

of others	1	2	3	4
3. You do a good job and get a poor evaluation	1	2	3	4
4. Someone makes a rule you don't like	1	2	3	4
5. People disagree with you	1	2	3	4
6. Your spouse (partner or significant other) gets angry and blows up at you for no good reason	1	2	3	4
7. Someone insults you or your family	1	2	3	4
8. Your spouse (partner or significant other) strongly criticizes you in front of family members	1	2	3	4
9. Someone cuts in front of you after you have been waiting in line for a long time	1	2	3	4
10. Your spouse (partner or significant other) criticizes you, or gets angry and blows up at you in a public place	1	2	3	4
11. You are under pressure or stress	1	2	3	4
12. You listen to someone talking and this person takes too long to come to the point	1	2	3	4
13. Your spouse (partner or significant other) walks away from you in the midst of a disagreement (discussion)	1	2	3	4

14. You are to meet someone
at a public place (street
corner,building, lobby,
restaurant) and the other
person is already 10 minutes
late   1   2   3   4

Total Points _____

Score yourself: Add up the points (1–4) for each item to get your total score, somewhere between 14 and 56. A person who scores 38 is just about average. If you score below 26, you are well down in the safe zone—not prone to become angry in a number of social situations. A score above 40 means that you may be a hothead—prone to respond to frustrating social situations with intense feelings of anger.

APPENDIX B: TAKE YOUR TEMPER TEST

The tests presented on the following pages—developed by Dr. Charles D. Spielberger and colleagues at the University of South Florida in Tampa—are widely used in research to determine the role of stress and emotions in health and psychological problems. You can use these tests to make a rough estimate of your characteristic way of coping with stress and the degree of stress present in your job.

Temper Test: Are You Stress Prone?

Directions: A number of statements that people have used to describe themselves are given below. Read each statement and then circle (or simply note in your mind) the answer that indicates how you generally feel. There are no right or wrong answers. Do not spend too much time on any one statement, but give the answer that seems to describe how you generally feel.

	Almost Never	Some times	Often	Almost Always
1.) I am quick tempered	1	2	3	4
2.) I feel annoyed when I am not given recognition for doing good work	1	2	3	4

3.)	I have a fiery temper	1	2	3	4
4.)	I feel infuriated when I do a good job and get a poor evaluation	1	2	3	4
5.)	I am a hotheaded person	1	2	3	4
6.)	It makes me furious when I am criticized in front of others	1	2	3	4
7.)	I get angry when I'm slowed down by others' mistakes	1	2	3	4
8.)	I fly off the handle	1	2	3	4
9.)	When I get mad, I say nasty things	1	2	3	4
10.)	When I get frustrated, I feel like hitting someone	1	2	3	4

Total Points   _____

Score Yourself: Add up the points (1–4) for each item to get your total score, somewhere between 10 and 40. A man who scores 17 or a woman who scores 18 is just about average. If you score below 13, you are well down in the safe zones, and perhaps unresponsive to situations that provoke others. But a score above 20 means you may be a hothead—scoring higher than three-quarters of those tested. (London, P. and Spielberger, C. D., Job Stress, hassles, and medical risk. Reprinted with permission from American Health 1983 March/April: 60.)

Job Stress Index: Are You Hassled?

Directions: This survey lists ten job-related events that have been identified as stressful by employees working in different settings. Please read each item and circle (or simply note in your mind) the answer that indicates the approximate number of times during the past month that you have been upset or bothered by each event.

<u>Number of Occurrences during Past Month</u>

1. I have been bothered
    by fellow workers not
    doing their job   0   1   2   3+

2. I have had inadequate
    support from my
    supervisor   0   1   2   3+

3. I have had problems
    getting along with my
    co-workers   0   1   2   3+

4. I have had trouble
    getting along with
    my supervisor   0   1   2   3+

5. I have felt pressed to
    make critical on-the-
    spot decisions   0   1   2   3+

6. I have been bothered
    by the fact that there
    aren't enough
    people to handle
    the job   0   1   2   3+

7. I have felt a lack of
    participation in
    policy decisions   0   1   2   3+

8. I have been con-
    cerned about my
    inadequate salary   0   1   2   3+

9. I have been troubled
    by a lack of recognition
    for good work   0   1   2   3+

10. I have been frustrated
    by excessive paperwork   0   1   2   3+

Total points   _____

    Score Yourself: To determine how your stress compares with other
workers, add up the points (0–3) that you circled for each item. Your
score will be between 0 and 30. Persons who score between 5 and 7 are
about average in how often they experience job-related stress. If you
score higher than 9, you may have cause for concern. At 4 or lower, you
have a relatively nonstressful job.

Double-Barreled Danger: 20+ and 9+

If you score higher than 20 on temper, and if your score is higher than 9
on the job stress index, you have a dangerous combination going.
Better cool yourself or the job. Double-digit job stress points to trouble,
especially if your personality runs high in irritability and temper.
Remember the double-barreled effect: If your personality makes you
anger prone, you have to watch out for jobs high in petty aggravations.
(London, P. and Spielberger, C.D., Job stress, hassles and medical risk.
Reprinted with permission from American Health 1983 March/April: 61.)

APPENDIX C: ANGER COPING STYLES ASSESSMENT

A number of different questionnaires have been used to determine how
people cope with and express feelings of anger. Two of these
questionnaires are presented on the following pages. You can use them
to make a rough determination of your usual way of coping with anger.

Questionnaire #1

    Directions: A few situations a person might face are presented
below. Please read each description and circle the appropriate number to
indicate how you would respond to the situation.

I.   Imagine that your spouse (partner) got angry and blew up at you
          at home about not having time for social activities.

          1. I would get angry or mad and show it.

          2. I would get angry or mad, but keep it in.

          3. I would try to stay calm and solve the problem with a
             discussion at a later time.

4. I would get annoyed, but would keep it in.

5. I would get annoyed and show it.

II.   Imagine that your spouse (partner) criticized you, or got angry and blew up at you in a public place. What would you do?

1. I would get angry or mad and show it.

2. I would get angry or mad, but keep it in.

3. I would try to stay calm and solve the problem with a discussion at a later time.

4. I would get annoyed, but would keep it in.

5. I would get annoyed and show it.

III.   Imagine that your spouse (partner) criticized you, got angry and blew up at you in front of your relatives. What would you do?

1. I would get angry or mad and show it.

2. I would get angry or mad, but keep it in.

3. I would try to stay calm and solve the problem with a discussion at a later time.

4. I would get annoyed, but would keep it in.

5. I would get annoyed and show it.

IV.   Imagine that your boss or supervisor got angry and blew up at you about your performance on a task (job) that you thought was good work. What would you do?

1. I would get angry or mad and show it.

2. I would get angry or mad, but keep it in.

3. I would try to stay calm and solve the problem with discussion at a later time.

4. I would get annoyed, but would keep it in.

  5. I would get annoyed and show it.

V.   Imagine that a cashier at a department store got angry and blew
       up at you for no apparent   reason. What would you do?

  1. I would get angry or mad and show it.

  2. I would get angry or mad, but keep it in.

  3. I would try to stay calm and solve the problem with a
     discussion at a later time.

  4. I would get annoyed, but would keep it in.

  5. I would get annoyed and show it.

     The first category or Anger-In (represented by choices 2 and 4)—
presumed to induce high blood pressure—is to ignore or walk away from
the conflict situation, leading to a static or declining-reality situation and
suppressed anger. The second coping category is Anger-Out
(represented by choices 1 and 5), expressing anger.to the attacker.
Although this circumvents suppression, over time it has questionable
results—in the worker's situation, particularly (i.e., the boss may react
punitively when attacked in return). A third category of response
represented by choice 3— perhaps the most controlled solution—is to
bypass anger, and manage to restore a fair situation by analysis of the
problem. This Anger-Reflection/Control category would seem to be
closer to the approach most favored for problem solving. The reflex
anger to an unfair attack is suppressed, but only because attention is
being directed at solving the problem associated with the unjust anger.
The calmer reflective approach toward the arbitrary use of power may, in
the long run, allow for mastery of stress.
     How consistent were your responses across the various situations?
Were you more likely to express your anger to your spouse (partner) at
home or in a public place? Were you more likely to express anger
outwardly to the cashier or your boss? Your responses probably show
that your manner or style of coping with anger varies depending on the
setting of the provocation (private versus public), and the status of the
attacker (cashier versus boss). A number of other factors (e.g., level of
anxiety, and fear about a counterattack) contribute to how you cope with
anger.

Questionnaire 2

Directions: Please circle the appropriate number that best describes how you and your spouse (partner) have handled tensions, disagreements, and other problems.

YOU

		Always	Most of the Time	Some of the Time	Hardly Ever	Never
1.	Initiated a discussion to air the problem	1	2	3	4	5
2.	Shouted or yelled	1	2	3	4	5
3.	Insulted your spouse (partner), called him/her names, or threatened him/her	1	2	3	4	5
4.	Kept distant from your spouse (partner)	1	2	3	4	5
5.	Gave in to your spouse (partner)	1	2	3	4	5
6.	Listened attentively to what your spouse (partner) was saying	1	2	3	4	5
7.	Tried to hide the tension or anger you felt	1	2	3	4	5
8.	Left the room or walked away from your spouse (partner) in the midst of a discussion	1	2	3	4	5
9.	Pushed, shoved, hit, or threw something at your spouse (partner)	1	2	3	4	5
10.	Refused to compromise	1	2	3	4	5

YOUR SPOUSE

		Most of the time	Some of the time	Hardly ever	Never
	Always				

1. Initiated a discussion to air the problem   1   2   3   4   5

2. Shouted or yelled   1   2   3   4   5

3. Insulted you, called you names, or threatened you   1   2   3   4   5

4. Kept distant from you   1   2   3   4   5

5. Gave in to you   1   2   3   4   5

6. Listened attentively to what you were saying   1   2   3   4   5

7. Tried to hide the tension or anger he/she felt   1   2   3   4   5

8. Left the room or walked away from you in the midst of a discussion   1   2   3   4   5

9. Pushed, shoved, hit, or threw something at you   1   2   3   4   5

10. Refused to compromise   1   2   3   4   5

Score Yourself: Add up the points (1–5) for questions 4, 5, 7, and 8 to obtain your ANGER-IN SCORE _____ If you score above 7, you are in the danger zone, more likely to suppress feelings of anger when you and your spouse (partner) have stress in your life. Remember the findings from the Tecumseh Community Health Project (see Chapter 1), which revealed that the mortality risk of those who suppress their anger is two times greater than those who express their anger.

To obtain your ANGER-OUT SCORE_____, add up the points for questions 2, 3, and 9. If you score above 5, you are in the danger zone and are probably in trouble with your spouse (partner) and yourself. There may be real reason for concern.

Your ANGER-REFLECTION SCORE_____ is obtained by adding up the points for questions 1 and 6. If you score below 5, you are in the safe zone and very responsive and understanding; but if you score below 3 on question 10, you are unable to compromise and come up with mutually satisfying solutions to problems with your spouse or partner.

How well do you know how your spouse (partner) copes with problems and stress? Are your coping styles similar?

Notes

INTRODUCTION

1. Tavris, C. <u>Anger: The Misunderstood Emotion</u>. New York: Simon and Schuster, 1982.

2. Lerner, H. G. <u>The Dance of Anger (A Woman's Guide to Changing the Patterns of Intimate Relationships)</u>. New York: Harper and Row, 1985.

1 ANGER, HOSTILITY, AND AGGRESSION: THE AHA! SYNDROME

1. Harburg E., Blakelock, E. H., and Roeper, P. J. Resentful and reflective coping with arbitrary authority and blood pressure: Detroit. <u>Psychosomatic Medicine</u> 1979, 3:189–202.

2. Spielberger, C. D. <u>Professional Manual for the State-Trait Anger Expression Inventory (STAXI)</u> (research ed.) Tampa, Fla.: Psychological Assessment Resources,1988.

3. Spielberger, C. D. and Butcher, J. N. (eds.). <u>Advances in Personality Assessment</u> , vol. 7. Hillsdale, N.J.: LEA, 1988.

4. Spielberger, C. D. and Krasner, S. S. The assessment of state and trait anxiety. In Burrows, G. D., Noyes, R., and Roth, M. (eds.), <u>Handbook of Anxiety,</u> vol. 2. Amsterdam: Elsevier Science Publishers, 1988.

5. Spielberger,C. D., Krasner, S. S., and Solomon, E. P. The

experience, expression, and control of anger. In Janisse, M. P. (ed.), Health Psychology: Individual Differences and Stress. New York: Springer Verlag, 1988.

6. Novaco, R . Anger Control: The Development and Evaluation of an Experimental Treatment. Lexington, Mass.: D.C. Heat Lexington Books,1975.

7. Schachter, S. and Singer, J. E. Cognitive, social, and physiological determinants of emotional state. Psychological Review 1962, 69:379–399.

8. Moyer, K. E. The Psychobiology of Aggression. New York: Harper and Row, 1976.

9. Buss, A. The Psychology of Aggression. New York: John Wiley and Sons, 1961.

10. Feshbach, S. Aggression. In: Mussen, P. H. (ed.), Carmichael's Manual of Child Psychology, vol 2. New York: Wiley, 1970.

11. Kaufman, H. Aggression and Altruism. New York: Holt, Rinehart, and Winston, 1970.

12. Spielberger, C. D., Johnson, E. H., Russell, S.F., Crane, R. J,. Jacobs, G. A., and Worden, T. The experience and expression of anger: Construction and validation of an anger expression scale. In Chesney, M. A. and Rosenman, R. (eds.), Anger and Hostility in Cardiovascular and Behavioral Disorders. Washington, D.C.: Hemisphere Publishing/McGraw-Hill, 1985.

13. Berkowitz, L. Is criminal violence normative behavior? Hostile and instrumental aggression and violent incidents. Journal of Research Crime and Delinquency, 1978, 15:148–161.

14. Moyer, K. E. The Psychology of Aggression. New York: Harper and Row, 1976.

15. Freud, S. Beyond the Pleasure Principle. New York: Boni and Liveright, 1927.

16. Klein, M. Contributions to Psychoanalysis. London: Hogarth Press, 1948.

17. Nunberg, H. Principles of Psychoanalysis. New York: International University Press, 1955.

18. Waelder, R. Critical discussion of the concept of an instinct of destruction. Bulletin of Philadelphia Association of Psychoanalysis 1956, 6:97–109.

19. Hartman, H., Kris, E., Lowenstein, R. Notes on the theory of aggression. Psychoanalytic Study of the Child 1949, 3:9-36.

20. Storr, A. Human Aggression. New York: Atheneum, 1968.

21. Fromm, E. Anatomy of Human Destructiveness. New York: Holt, Rinehart, and Winston, 1973.

22. Horney, K. Our Inner Conflicts. New York: Norton, 1945.

23. Saul, L. J. The Hostile Mind. New York: Random House, 1956.

24. Dollard, J., Doob, L. W., Miller, N. E., Mowrer, O. H., and Sears, R. R. Frustration and Aggression. New Haven, Conn.: Yale University Press, 1939.

25. Breuer, J. and Freud, S. Studies on Hysteria. Translated by James Strachey. New York: Basic Books, 1982.

26. Freud, S. Why war? In Strachey, J. (ed.), Collected Papers, vol. 5 London: Hogarth Press, 1959, (originally published 1933).

27. Berkowitz, L. Aggressive cues in aggressive behavior and hostility catharsis. Psychological Review, 1964, 71:104–22.

28. Brown, J. S. and Farber, I.E. Emotions conceptualized as intervening variables with suggestions toward a theory of frustration. Psychological Bulletin 1951 48:465–95; reprinted in Psychosomatic Medicine 1989, 51:249.

29. Hokanson, J. E., Burgess, M., and Cohen, M. Effects of displaced aggression on systolic blood pressure. Journal of Abnormal and Social Psychology 1963, 67:214–18.

30. Hokanson, J. E. and Shelter, S. The effect of overt aggression on physiological arousal level. Journal of Abnormal and Social Psychology 1961, 63:446–48.

31. Baker, J. W. and Schair, K. W. Effects of aggressing "alone" or

"with others" on physiological and psychological arousal. <u>Journal of Personality and Social Psychology</u> 1969, 12:80–86.

32. Gambaro, S. and Rabin, A. I.   Diastolic blood pressure responses following direct and displaced aggression after anger arousal in high and low guilt subjects. <u>Journal of Personality and Social Psychology</u> 1969, 12(1):87–94.

33. Van Egeren, L. Cardiovascular changes during social competition in a mixed-motive game. <u>Journal of Personality and Social Psychology</u> 1979, 37:858–64.

34. Arnold, M. B. (eds.) <u>Feelings and Emotions</u>. New York: Academic Press, 1970.

35. Lazarus, R. and Folkman, S. Coping and adaptation. In Gentry, W. D. (ed.), <u>Handbook of Behavioral Medicine</u>. New York: Guilford Press, 1984.

36. Lazarus, R. S. and Folkman, S. <u>Stress, Appraisal, and Coping</u>. New York: Springer, 1984.

37. Buss, A. H. and Plomin, R. A. <u>A Temperament Theory of Personality Development</u>. London: John Wiley and Sons, 1975.

38. Smith, T. W., McGonigle, M., Turner, C. W., Ford, M. H. and Slattery, M. L. Cynical hostility in adult male twins. Abstract of the 1989 American Psychosomatic Medicine Society Meeting.

39. Buss, A. H. and Durkee, A.   An inventory for assessing different kinds of hostility. <u>Journal of Consulting Psychology</u> 1957 21:343–49.

40. Mathews, K. A. and Woodall, K. L. Childhood origins of overt Type A behavior and cardiovascular reactivity to behavioral stressors. <u>Annals of Behavioral Medicine</u> 1988, vol. 10:71–77.

41. Rosenman, R. H. Health consequences of anger and implications for treatment. In Chesney, M. A., and Rosenman, R. H. (eds.), <u>Anger and Hostility in Cardiovascular and Behavioral Disorders</u>. Washington, D..C.: Hemisphere Publishing/McGraw-Hill, 1985.

42. Friedman, M. and Rosenman, R. <u>Type-A Behavior and Your Heart</u>. New York: Knopf, 1974.

43. Blumenthal, J., Williams, R. B., Kong, Y., Schanberg, S. M. and

Thompson, T. W. Type-A behavior patterns and coronary atherosclerosis. Circulation 1978, 58:634–39.

44. Williams, R., Barefoot, J. C., Shekelle. R. B. The health consequences of hostility. In Chesney, M. A. and Rosenman, R. H. (eds.), Anger and Hostility in Cardiovascular and Behavioral Disorders. Washington, D.C.: Hemisphere Publishing/McGraw-Hill 1985.

45.Williams, R. B. The Trusting Heart. New York: Times Books Random House, New York, 1989.

46. Shekelle, R. B., Gale, M., Ostfeld, M. A., and Paul, O. Hostility, risk of CHD, and mortality. Psychosomatic Medicine 1983, 45:109–14.

47. Barefoot, J. C., Dahlstrom, W. S., and Williams, R. B. Jr. Hostility, CHD incidence, and total mortality: A 25-year follow-up study of 255 physicians. Psychosomatic Medicine 1983 45:59–63.

48. McCranie, E., Watkins, L., Brandsma, J., and Sisson, B. Hostility, coronary heart disease (CHD) incidence, and total mortality: Lack of association in a 25 year follow-up study of 478 physicians. Journal of Behavioral Medicine 1986, 9:119–25.

49. Smith, T. W. and Frohn, K.D. What's so unhealthy about hostility? Construct validity and psychosocial correlates of the Cook and Medley Ho scale. Health Psychology 1985, 4: 503-520.

50. Johnson, E. H. and Gant, L. Emotional and psychosomatic reactions related to suppressed (anger-in) and expressed (anger-out) anger. Unpublished manuscript, University of Michigan Medical Center, Ann Arbor, 1989.

51. Julius, M., Harburg, E., Cottington, E., and Johnson, E. H. Anger-coping types, blood pressure, and total mortality: A follow-up in Tecumseh, Michigan, 1971–1983. American Journal of Epidemiology 1986, 124:220–33.

52. Julius, S., Schork, N., Johnson, E. H., Jones, K., Krause. L,. and Nazzaro, P. Independence of pressure reactivity from blood pressure levels in Tecumseh, Michigan. Hypertension, in press.

53. Julius, S., Mejia, A., Jones, K., Krause, L., Schork, N., van de Ven, C,. Johnson, E. H., Petrin, J., Sekkarie, A,. Kjeldsen, S. E., Schmouder, R., Gupta, R., Ferraro, J,. Nazzaro, P., and Weissfeld, J. "White coat" versus "sustained" borderline hypertension in Tecumseh, Michigan. Hypertension, in press.

54. Julius, M., Harburg, E., and Cottington, E. Martial pair anger-coping types and all cause mortality in Tecumseh (1971–1983 follow-up). Paper presented at the Gerontological Society of America 39th Annual Scientific Meeting, Chicago, November 19–23, 1986.

55. Koskenvuo, M., Kaprio, J,. Rose, R. J,. Kesniemi, A., Sarna, S., Heikkil, K., and Langinvainio, H. Hostility as a risk factor for mortality and ischemic heart disease. Psychosomatic Medicine 1988, 50(4):330–40.

56. Dembroski, T., MacDougall, J. M., Williams, R. B., Haney, T. L. and Blumenthal, J. A. Components of Type A behavior, hostility, and anger-in: relationship to angiographic findings. Psychosomatic Medicine 1985, 47:219–33.

2   THE ROLE OF THE AHA! SYNDROME IN HEALTH AND
     PSYCHOLOGICAL WELL-BEING

1.Williams, R. B. The Trusting Heart. New York:Times Books Random House, 1989.

2. Kalbak, K. Incidence of atherosclerosis in patients with rheumatoid arthritis receiving long-term corticosteroid therapy. Annals of Rheumatic Disease 1972, 31:196–200.

3. Troxler, R. G., Sprague, E. A., Albanese, R. A., et al. The association of elevated plasma
cortisol and early atherosclerosis as demonstrated by coronary angiography. Atherosclerosis 1977, 26:151–62.

4. Klaiber, E. L., Broverman, D. M., Haffajee, C. I. et al. Serum-estrogen levels in men with acute myocardial-infarction. American Journal of Medicine 1982, 73:872–81.

5. Luria, M. H., Johnson, M. W., Pego, R., Secu, C. A., Manubens, D. J., Wieland, M. K., and Wieland, R. G. Relationship b/w sex hormones, myocardial infarction, and occlusive coronary disease. Archives of Internal Medicine 1982, 142:42–44.

6. Phillips, G. B., Kastelli, W. P., Abbott, R. D., and McNamara, P. M. Association of hyperestogenemia and coronary heart disease in men in the Framingham cohort. American Journal of Medicine 1983, 74:863–69.

7. Graves, P. I., and Thomas, C. B. Themes of interaction in medical student's Rorschach responses and predictors of mid-life health or disease. Psychosomatic Medicine 1981, 43:215–26.

8. Dorian, B., Garfinkel, P., Keystone, E., Gorczynski, R., Darby P and Garner D. Occupational stress and immunity (abstract). Psychosomatic Medicine 1985, 47:77.

9. Kiecolt-Glaser, J. K., Glaser, R., Strain, E. C., Stout, J. C., Tarr, K. L., Holiday, J. E. and Speicher, C. E. Modulation of cellular immunity in medical students. Journal of Behavioral Medicine 1984, 9:5–21.

10. Kiecolt-Glaser, J. K., Garner, R., Speicher, E. C., Penn, G. and Glaser, R. Psychosocial modifiers of immunocompetence in medical students. Psychosomatic Medicine 1984, 46:7–14.

11. Baker, G. B. H. Psychological factors and immunity. Invited review. Journal of Psychosomatic Research 1987, 31:1–10.

12. Cannon, W. B. Bodily Changes in Pain, Hunger, Fear, and Rage. New York: Appleton-Century, 1929.

13. Abraham, K. Selected Papers of Karl Abraham. London: Hogarth Press and Institute of Psychoanalysis, 1927, pp.137–56.

14. Seligman, M. Helplessness: On Depression, Development, and Death. San Francisco: W.H. Freeman, 1975.

15. Abramson, L. Y., Seligman, M. E. P. and Teasdale, J. D. Learned helplessness in humans: Critique and reformulation. Journal of Abnormal Psychology 1978, 87:49–74.

16. Peterson, C., Seligman, M., Vaillant, G. Pessimistic explanatory style is a risk factor for physical illness: A thirty-five year longitudinal study. Journal of Personality and Social Psychology 1988, 55:23–27.

17. Wender, P. H. and Klein, D. F. Mind, Mood, and Medicine: A Guide to the New Biopsychiatry. New York: Farrar, Straus, and Giroux, 1981.

18. Johnson, E. H. and Gant, L. Emotional and psychosomatic reactions related to suppressed (anger-in) and expressed (anger-out) anger. Unpublished manuscript, University of Michihan Medical Center, Ann Arbor, 1989.

19. Jackson, J., Tucker, B., and Bowman, P. H. Conceptual and Methodological Problems in Minority Research. Ann Arbor:University of Michigan, Pacific/Asian American Mental Health Research Center, 1982; pp. 5–29.

20. Johnson, E. H., Broman, C. L. The relationship of anger expression to health problems in a national survey. Journal of Behavioral Medicine 1987, 10:103–16.

21. Broman, C. L. and Johnson, E. H. Anger expression and life stress among blacks: Their role in physical health. Journal of the National Medical Association 1988, 80:1329–34.

22. Harburg, E., Blakelock, E. H. and Roeper, P. J. Resentful and reflective coping with arbitrary authority and blood pressure: Detroit. Psychosomatic Medicine 1979, 3:189–202.

23. Gentry, W. D. Relationship of anger-coping styles and blood pressure among black Americans. In Chesney, M. A. and Rosenman, R. H. (eds.), Anger and Hostility in Cardiovascular and Behavioral Disorders. Washington, D.C.: Hemisphere Publishing/McGraw-Hill, 1985.

24. Kennedy, C. D., Chesney, A. P., Gentry, W. D., Gary, H. E. and Harburg, E. Anger-coping style as a mediator in the relationship between hostility and blood pressure. Unpublished manuscript 1984.

25. Chesney, A. P., Gentry, W. D., Gary, H. E., Kennedy, C. and Harburg, E. Anger-coping style as a mediator in the relationship between life strain and blood pressure. Unpublished manuscript 1984.

26. Selye, H. Stress in Health and Disease. New York: Butterworth, 1976.

27. Funkenstein, D. H., King, S., and Drolette, M. Mastery of Stress. Cambridge, Mass: Harvard University Press, 1957.

28. Siegel, J. Anger in cardiovascular risk in adolescents. Health Psychology 1984, 3:293–313.

29. Tavris, C. Anger: The Misunderstood Emotion. New York: Simon and Schuster, 1982.

30. Novaco, R. W. Anger and its therapeutic regulation. In Chesney, M. A. and Rosenman, R. H. (eds.), Anger and Hostility in Cardiovascular and Behavioral Disorders. Washington, D.C.:Hemisphere Publishing/McGraw-Hill, 1985.

31. Patterson, G. R. A microsocial analysis of anger and irritable behavior. In Chesney, M. A. and Rosenman, R. H. (eds.), <u>Anger and Hostility in Cardiovascular and Behavioral Disorders</u>.Washington, D.C.: Hemisphere Publishing/McGraw-Hill, 1985.

32. Harburg, E., Erfurt, J. C., Hauenstein, L. S., Chape, C., Schull, W. J., and Schork, M. A. Socioecological stress, suppressed hostility, skin color, and black–white male blood pressure: Detroit. <u>Psychosomatic Medicine</u> 1973, 35:276–96.

33. Novaco, R. W. Anger Control: <u>The Development and Evaluation of an Experimental Treatment</u>. Lexington, Mass.:D.C. Heath Lexington Books, 1975.

34. Megargee, E. The dynamics of aggression and their application to cardiovascular disorders. In Chesney, M. A. and Rosenman, R. H. (eds.), <u>Anger and Hostility in Cardiovascular and Behavioral Disorders</u>. Washington, D.C.: Hemisphere Publishing/McGraw-Hill, 1985.

35. Averill, J. R. <u>Anger and Aggression: An Essay on Emotion</u>. New York: Springer Verlag, 1982.

3   CARDIOVASCULAR DISEASE AND THE AHA! SYNDROME

1. Dunbar, H. F. Hypertensive cardiovascular disease. In Dunbar, H. F. (ed.), <u>Psychosomatic Diagnosis</u>. New York: Hoebar, 1943.

2. Alexander, F. Emotional factors in essential hypertension: Presentation of a tentative hypothesis. <u>Psychosomatic Medicine</u> 1939, 1:175–79.

3. Alexander, F. <u>Psychosomatic Medicine: Its Principles and Application</u>, New York:W. W. Norton, 1987. (Originally published in 1948).

4. Diamond, E. L. The role of anger and hostility in essential hypertension and coronary heart disease. <u>Psychological Bulletin</u> 1982, 92: 410–33.

5. Gentry, W. D., Chesney, A. P., Gary, H. G., Hall, R. D., and Harburg, E. Habitual anger-coping styles. I. Effect on mean blood pressure and risk for essential hypertension. <u>Psychosomatic Medicine</u> 1982, 44:273–81.

6. Gentry, W. D. Relationship of anger-coping styles and blood pressure among black Americans. In Chesney, M. A. and Rosenman, R. H. (eds.), <u>Anger and Hostility in Cardiovascular and Behavioral Disorders</u>. Washington, D.C.:Hemesphere Publishig/McGraw-Hill, 1985.

7. Herd, J. A. Cardiovascular Disease and Hypertension. In Gentry. W. D. (Ed.), <u>Handbook of Behavioral Medicine</u>. New York: Guilford Press, 1984.

8. Julius, S., Bassett, D. R. (eds.). <u>Handbook of Hypertension</u> vol. 9: <u>Behavioral Factors in Hypertension.</u> Amsterdam: Elsevier Science Publisher, 1987.

9. Cannon, W. <u>The Wisdom of the Body</u>. New York: Norton, 1932.

10. Saul, L. J. Hostility in cases of essential hypertension. <u>Psychosomatic Medicine</u> 1939, 1:1.

11. Ayman, D. Personality type of patients with arteriolar essential hypertension. <u>American Journal of Medical Science</u> 1933, 186:213–23.

12. Cochrane, R. Hostility and neuroticism among unselected essential hypertensives. <u>Journal of Psychosomatic Research</u> 1973, 17:215–18.

13. Kidson, M. A. Personality and hypertension. <u>Journal of Psychosomatic Research</u> 1973, 17:35.

14. Matarazzo, J. D. An experimental study of aggression in the hypertensive patient. <u>Journal of Personality</u> 1954, 22:423–47.

15. Harburg, E., Erfurt, J. C., Hausenstein, L.S., Chape, C., Schull, W. J., and Schork, M. A. Socio-ecological stress, suppressed hostility, skin color, and black-white male blood pressure: Detroit. <u>Psychosomatic Medicine</u> 1973, 35:276–96.

16. Johnson, E. H. Anger and anxiety as determinants of elevated blood pressure in adolescents: The Tampa Study. Ph.D. dissertation, Department of Psychology, University of South Florida, Tampa, 1984.

17. Johnson, E. H., Spielberger, C. D., Worden, T. J., and Jacobs, G. Emotional and familial determinants of elevated blood pressure in black and white adolescent males. <u>Journal of Psychosomatic Research</u> 1987, 31:287–300.

18. Johnson, E. H., Schork, N. and Spielberger, C. D. Emotional

and familial determinants of elevated blood pressure in black and white adolescent females. Journal of Psychosomatic Research 1987, 31:731–41.

19. Johnson, E. H. Interrelationship between psychological factors, overweight, and blood pressure in adolescents. Journal of Adolescent Health Care 1990, 11:310–318.

20. Schneider, R., Egan, B., Johnson, E. H., Drobney, H. and Julius, S. Anger and anxiety in borderline hypertension. Psychosomatic Medicine 1986, 48:242–48.

21. Johnson, E. H . Cardiovascular reactivity, emotional factors, and home blood pressure in black males with and without a parental history of hypertension. Psychosomatic Medicine 1989, 51:390–403.

22. Cottington, E., Brock, B. M., House, J. S., and Hawthorn, V. M. Psychosocial factors and blood pressure in the Michigan Statewide Blood Pressure Survey. American Journal of Epidemiology 1985, 121:515–29.

23. Cobb, S. and Rose, R. M. Hypertension, peptic ulcers, and diabetes in air traffic controllers. Journal of the American Medical Association 1973, 224:489–92.

24. Rose, R. M. Endocrine responses to stressful psychological events. Psychiatric Clinics of North America 1980, 3:1–15.

25. Reynolds, R. C. Community and occupational influences in stress at Cape Kennedy: relationship to Heart Disease. In Eliot, R. S. (ed.), Stress and the Heart. Mt. Kisco, N.Y.: Futura, 1974.

26. van Dijkhuizen, N., Reicher, H. Psychosocial stress in industry: A heartache for middle management? Psychotherapy Psychosomatics 1980, 34:124–34.

27. Aro, S. Occupational stress, health-related behavior, and blood pressure: A 5-year follow-up. Preventive Medicine 1984, 13:333–48.

28. Mathews, K. A,. Cottington, E. M., Talbott, E., Kuller, L. H. and Siegel, J. M. Stressful work conditions and diastolic blood pressure among blue-collar factory workers. American Journal of Epidemiology 1987, 126:280–91.

29. House, J. S., McMichael, A. J., Wells, J. A., Kaplan, B. H., and

Landerman, L. R. Occupational stress and health among factory workers. Journal of Health and Social Behavior 1979, 20:139–60.

30. House, J. Barriers to work stress: I. Social support. In Gentry, W. D., Benson, H. and de Wolff, C. (eds.), Behavioral Medicine: Work, Stress, and Health. The Hague: Martinus Nijhoff, 1984.

31. Kasl, S. V. and Cobb, S. Blood pressure changes in men undergoing job loss: A preliminary report. Psychosomatic Medicine 1970, 32:19–38.

32. Cottingtom, E. M. Occupational stress, psychosocial modifiers, and blood pressure in a blue-collar population. Ph.D. dissertation, University of Pittsburgh, Graduate School of Public Health, 1983.

33. Cottington, E. M., Mathews, K. A,. Talbott, E., and Kuller, L. H. Occupational stress, suppressed anger, and hypertension. Psychosomatic Medicine 1986, 48:249–60.

34. Manuck, S., Morrison, R. L., Bellack, A. S., and Polefrone, J. M. Behavioral factors in hypertension: Cardiovascular responsivity, anger, and social competence. In Chesney, M. A., Rosenman, R. H. (eds.), Anger and Hostility in Cardiovascular and Behavioral Disorders. Washington, D.C.:Hemisphere Publishing/McGraw-Hill, 1985.

35. Manuck, S. B. and Proietti, J. Parental hypertension and cardiovascular response to cognitive isometric challenge. Psychophysiology 1982, 19:481–89.

36. Keane, T. M., Martin, J. E., Berler, E. S., Wooten, L. S., Fleece, E. L., and Williams, J. G. Are hypertensives less assertive? A controlled evaluation. Journal of Consulting and Clinical Psychology 1982, 50:499–508.

37. Linden, W. and Fauerstein, M. Essential hypertension and social coping behavior. Journal of Human Stress 1981, 7:28–34.

38. Goldstein, D. S., Plasma catecholamines and essential hypertension: An analytical review. Hypertension 1983, 5 86–99.

39. Goldstein, D. S. Plasma norepinephrine in essential hypertension: A study of studies. Hypertension 1981, 3:48–52.

40. Julius S, Schork N, and Schork MA. Sympathetic hyperactivity in early stages of hypertension: The Ann Arbor data set.Journal of Cardiovascular Pharmacology 1988, 12 (Suppl. 3):S121–29.

41. Esler, M., Julius, S., Randall, O., Harburg, E., Gardiner, H., and DeQuattro, V. Mild high-renin essential hypertension: Neurogenic human hypertension? New England Journal of Medicine 1977, 296:405–11.

42. Julius, S., Schneider, R., and Egan, B. Suppressed anger in hypertension: Facts and problems. In Chesney, M. A. and Rosenman, R. H. (eds.), Anger and Hostility in Cardiovascular and Behavioral Disorders. Washington, D.C.: Hemisphere Publishing/McGraw-Hill,1985.

43. DeQuattro, V., Sullivan, P., Foti, A., Schoentgen, S., Kolloch, R., Verasales, G., and Levine, D. Central neurogenic mechanisms in hypertension and in postural hypotension. In Laragh, J,. Buhler, F., and Seldin, D. (eds.), Frontiers in Hypertension Research. New York: Springer-Verlag, 1981.

44. Perini, C., Muller, F. B., Rauchfleisch, U., and Buhler, F. Hyperadrenergic borderline hypertension is characterized by suppressed aggression. Journal of Cardiovascular Pharmacology 1986, 8 (Suppl 5):53.

45. Krantz, D. S. and Manuck, S. B. Acute psychophysiologic reactivity and risk of cardiovascular disease: A review and methodologic critique. Psychological Bulletin 1984, 96:435–64.

46. Julius, S. and Johnson, E. H. Stress, autonomic hyperactivity, and essential hypertension: An enigma. Journal of Hypertension 1985, 3:11–17.

47. Falkner, B., Onesti, G., Angelakos, E. T., Fernandes, M. and Langman, C. Cardiovascular response to mental stress in normal adolescents with hypertensive parents: Hemodynamics and mental stress in adolescents. Hypertension 1979, 1: 23-30.

48. Falkner, B., Onesti, G., and Hamstra, B. Stress response characteristics of adolescents with high genetic risk for essential hypertension: A five-year follow-up. Clinical and Experimental Genetic Hypertension 1981, 3:583–91.

49. Sokolow, M., Werdegar, D., Kain, H. K., Hinman, A. T. Relationship between level of blood pressure measured casually and by portable recorders and severity of complications in essential hypertension. Circulation 1966, 34:279–98.

50. Perloff, D., Sokolow, M. and Gowan, R. The prognostic value

of ambulatory blood pressure. Journal of the American Medical Association 1983, 249:2792–98.

51. Johnson, E. H. and Egan, B. M. Ambulatory blood pressure monitoring: Is it worth it? Cardio, September 1988, 5:95–114.

52. Kleinert, H. D., Harshfield, G. A., Pickering, T. G., Devereux, R. B., Sullivan, P. A., Mallory, W. K., and Laragh, J. H. What is the value of home blood pressure measurement in patients with mild hypertension? Hypertension 1984, 7:574–78.

53. Pickering, T. G., Harshfield, G. A., Devereux, R. B. and Laragh, J. H. What is the role of ambulatory blood pressure monitoring in the management of hypertensive patients? Hypertension 1985, 7:171–77.

54. Van Egeren, L. F. and Madarasmi, S. A computer-assisted diary (CAD) for ambulatory blood pressure monitoring. American Journal of Hypertension 1988, 1:179S–85S.

55. Devereux, R. B., Pickering, T. G., Harshfield, G. A., Kleinert, H. D., Denby, L., Clark, L., Pregibon, D., Jason, M., Kleiner, B. Borer, J. S. and Laragh, J. H. Left ventricular hypertrophy in patients with hypertension: importance of blood pressure response to regularly recurring stress. Circulation 1983, 68:470–76.

56. Drayer, J. I. M., Weber, M. A. and DeYoung, J. L. Blood pressure as a determinant of cardiac left ventricular muscle mass. Archives of Internal Medicine 1983, 143:90–92.

57. Kaplan, N. W. and Stamler, J. Prevention of Coronary Heart Disease. Philadelphia: W. B. Saunders, 1983.

58. Kaplan, N. W. Prevent Your Heart Attack. New York: Charles Scribner's Sons, 1982.

59. Keys, A., Aravanis, C., Blackburn, H., van Buchem, F. G. P., Buzima, R., Djordevic, B. X., Fidanza, F., Karvonen, M. J,. Nenotti, A., Puddu, V., and Taylor, H. L. Probability of middle-aged men developingcoronary heart disease in five years. Circulation 1972, 45:815–28.

60. Haynes, S. G., Levine, S., Scotch, N., Feinleib, M,. and Kannel, W. B. The relationship of psychosocial factors to coronary heart disease in the Framingham Study. II. Prevalence of coronary heart disease. American Journal of Epidemiology 1987, 167:384–402.

61. Friedman, M. and Rosenman, R. Type-A Behavior and Your Heart. New York: Knopf, 1974.

62. Haynes, S,. Feinleib, M., Levine, S., Scotch, N., and Kannel, W. B. The relationship of psychosocial factors to coronary heart disease in the Framingham Study. I. Methods and risk factors. American Journal of Epidemiology 1978, 167:362–83.

63. Osler, W . Lectures on Angina and Allied States. New York: Appleton, 1982.

64. Menninger, K. A.and Menninger, W. C . Psychoanalytic observations in cardiac disorders. American Heart Journal 1936, 11:10–21.

65. Rosenman, R. H., Friedman, M., Straus, R., Wurm, M,. Kositchek, R., Hahn, W., and Wethessen, N. T. A predictive study of coronary heart disease: The Western Collaborative Group Study. Journal of the American Medical Association 1964 189:15–22.

66. Rosenman, R. H., Brand, R. J., Sholtz, R. I., and Friedman, M. Multivariate prediction of coronary heart disease during 8.5 year follow-up in the Western Collaborative Group Study. American Journal of Cardiology 1976, 37:903–10.

67. Review Panel on Coronary-prone Behavior and Coronary Heart Disease. Coronary-prone behavior and coronary heart disease: A critical review. Circulation 1981, 63:1199–1215.

68. Dimsdale, J. A perspective on Type-A behavior and coronary heart disease. New England Journal of Medicine 1988, 318:110–12.

69. Belgian-French Pooling Project. Assessment of Type A behavior by the Bortner scale and ischemic heart disease. European Heart Journal 1984, 5:440º–46.

70. Shekelle, R. B., Hulley, S. B., Neaton, J. D., Billings, J. H., Borhani, N. O., Gerace, T. A,. Jacobs, D. R., Lasser, N. L., Mittlemark, M. B., and Stamler, J., for the Multiple Risk Factor Intervention Trial Research Group. The MRFIT behavior pattern study. II. Type A behavior and incidence of coronary heart disease. American Journal of Epidemiology 1985, 122:559–70.

71. Ruberman, W., Weinblatt, E., Goldberg, J. D., and Chaudbury, B. Psychosocial influence on mortality after myocardial infarction. New England Journal of Medicine 1984, 311 552–59.

72. Scherwitz, L., McKelvain, R., Lamon, C., Patterson, J., Dutton, L., Yusin, S., Lester, J,. Kraft, I., Rochelle, D., and Leachman, R. Type A behavior, self-involvement, and coronary atherosclerosis. Psychosomatic Medicine 1983, 45:47–58.

73. Ragland, D. and Brand, R. Type-A behavior and mortality from coronary heart disease. New England Journal of Medicine 1988, 318:65–69.

74. Matthews, K., Glass, D., Rosenman, R., and Raymond, B. Competitive drive, pattern A, and coronary heart disease: A further analysis of some data from the Western Collaborative Group Study. Journal of Chronic Disease 1977, 30:489–98.

75. Chesney, M. Anger and Hostility: Future Implications for Behavioral Medicine. In Chesney, M. A. and Rosenman, R. H. (eds.), Anger and Hostility in Cardiovascular and Behavioral Disorders. Washington, D.C.: Hemisphere Publishing/McGraw-Hill, 1985.

76. Dembroski, T. M,. MacDougall, J. M., Williams, R. B,. Haney, T. L., and Blumenthal, J. A. Components of Type A behavior, hostility, and anger-in: Relationship to angiographic findings. Psychosomatic Medicine 1985, 47:219–33.

77. Dembroski, T. M., MacDougall, J. M., Herd, J. A., and Shields, J. L. Effects of level of challenge on pressor and heart responses in Type A and B subjects. Journal of Applied Social Psychology 1979, 9:209–28.

78. Dembroski, T. M., MacDougall, J. M., Shields, J. L., Petitto, J., and Lushene, R. Components of Type A coronary-prone behavior pattern and cardiovascular responses to psychomotor challenge. Journal of Behavioral Medicine 1978, 1:159–76.

79. Diamond, E. L., Schneiderman, N., Schwartz, D., Smith, J. C., Vorp, R., and Pasin, R. D. Harassment, hostility, and Type A as determinants of cardiovascular reactivity during competition. Journal of Behavioral Medicine 1984, 7:171–89.

80. Camargo, C., Vranizan, K. M., Thoresen, C. E., and Wood, P. D. Type A Behavior Pattern and Alcohol Intake in Middle-Aged Men. Psychosomatic Medicine 1986, 48:575–80.

81. Weidner, G., Sexton, G., McLellarn, R., Connor, S. L., and Matarazzo, J. D. The role of Type A behavior and hostility in an elevation

of plasma lipids in adult women and men. Psychosomatic Medicine 1987, 49:136–45.

82. Grundy, S. and Winston, M. American Heart Association Low-Fat, Low-Cholesterol Cookbook, New York: Times Books/Random House, 1989.

83. Becker, G. L. Heart Smart. Fireside, 1987.

84. Kowalski, R. E. The 8-Week Cholesterol Cure. New York: Harper and Row, 1989.

85. King, P. Double jeopardy: Cholesterol and Type A. Minding your health—Mind over cholesterol. Psychology Today, 1989, Septembe:26.

86. Chollar, S. Hidden emotion, high Cholesterol. Minding your health—Mind over cholesterol. Psychology Today, 1989, September:24.

87. Lundberg, U., Hedman, M., Melin, B., and Frankenhaeuser, M. Type A behavior in healthy males and females as related to physiological reactivity and blood lipids. Psychosomatic Medicine 1989, 51:113–22.

88. Waldstein, S. R., Manuck, S. B. Bachen, E. A., Muldoon, M. F., and Bricker, P. L. Anger expression, lipids, and lipoproteins. Poster presentation, At the Eleventh Annual Meeting of the Society of Behavioral Medicine, April 18–20, 1990, Chicago, p. 102, Session Abstract.

4 CANCER, ULCERS, SMOKING, AND PSORIASIS

1. LeShan, L. The Medium, the Mystic, and the Physicist. New York: Viking Press, 1975.

2. Thomas, C. B. and Duszynski, K. R. Closeness to parents and the family constellation in a prospective study of five disease states: Suicide, mental illness, malignant tumor,hypertension, and coronary heart disease. Johns Hopkins Medical Journal 1974, 134:251–70.

3. Thomas, C. B., Duszynski, K. R., and Shaffer, J. W. Family attitudes reported in youth as potential predictors of cancer Psychosomatic Medicine 1979, 41:287–302.

4. Graves, P. L. and Thomas, C. B. Themes of interaction in

medical students' Rorschach responses as predictors of midlife health or disease. Psychosomatic Medicine 1981, 43:215–25.

5. Graves, P. L., Mean, L. A., and Pearson, T. A. The Rorschach interaction scale as a potential predictor of cancer. Psychosomatic Medicine 1986, 48:549–63.

6. Green, W. A. The psychosocial setting of the development of leukemia and lymphoma. Annals of the New York Academy of Sciences 1966, 125:794–801.

7. Kissen, D. Psychological factors, personality and lung cancer in men aged 55–64. British Journal of Medical Psychology 1967, 40:29–43.

8. Greer, S. and Morris, T. Psychological attitudes of women who develop breast cancer: A controlled study. Journal of Psychosomatic Research 1975, 19:147–53.

9. Greer, S., Morris, T., and Pettingale, K. W. Psychological response to breast cancer: effect on outcome. Lancet 1979, 2:785–87.

10. Pettingale, K. W., Morris, T., Greer, S., and Haybittle, J. L. Mental attitudes to cancer: An additional prognostic factor. Lancet 1985, 1:750.

11. Pettingale, K. W., Greer, S., and Tee, D. E. H. Serum IgA and emotional expression in breast cancer patients. Journal of Psychosomatic Research 1977, 21:395–99.

12. Pettingale, K. W., Burgess, C., and Greer, S. Psychological response to cancer diagnosis—I. Correlations with prognostic variables. Journal of Psychosomatic Research 1988, 32:255–62.

13. Burgess, C., Morris, T., and Pettingale, K.W. Psychological response to cancer diagnosis- II. Evidence for coping styles (coping styles and cancer diagnosis). Journal of Psychosomatic Research 1988, 32:263–72.

14. Temoshok, L., VanDyke, C., and Zegous, L. S. (eds.), Emotions in Health and Illness. New York: Grune and Stratton, 1983.

15. Kneier, A. W. and Temoshok, L. Repressive coping reactions in patients with malignant melanoma as compared to cardiovascular patients. Journal of Psychosomatic Research 1984, 28:145–55.

16. Heisel, J. S,. Locke, S. E., Kraus, L. J., and Williams, R. M. Natural killer cell activity and MMPI scores of a cohort of college students. American Journal Psychiatry 1986, 143:1382–86.

17. Levy, S. M. Presentation at the Society for Behavioral Medicine, 7th Annual Scientific Sessions, San Francisco, March 5–8, 1986.

18. Grossarth-Maticek, R., Bastiaans, J., and Kanazir, D. T. Psychosocial factors as strong predictors of mortality from cancer, ischemic heart disease, and stroke: The Yugoslav prospective study. Journal of Psychosomatic Research 1985, 29:167–76.

19. Eysenck, H. J. Personality, stress, and cancer: Prediction and prophylaxis. British Journal of Medical Psychology, 1988, 61:57–75.

20. Grossarth-Maticek, R., Eysenck, H. J., and Vetter H, Schmidt P. Psychological types and chronic disease. Results of the Heidelberg Prospective Psychosomatic Intervention Study. Paper presented at the International Conference on Health Psychology at Tilburg University The Netherlands, July 1986.

21. Persky, V., Kempthorne-Rowe, J. R., and Shekelle, R. Personality and risk of cancer: 20-Year follow-up of a Western Electric Study. Psychosomatic Medicine 1987, 49:435–49.

22. Blumberg, E. M., West ,P. M., and Ellis, F. W. A possible relationship between psychological factors and human cancer. Psychosomatic Medicine 1954, 16:227–86.

23. Baker, G. B. H. Psychological factors and immunity. Invited review. Journal of Psychosomatic Research 1987, 31:1–10.

24. Melnechuk, T. Emotions, Brain, Immunity and Health: A Review. In Clynes, M. and Panksepp, J. (eds.), Emotions and Psychopathology. New York and London: Plenum Press, 1988.

25. Kiecolt-Glaser, J. F., Fisher, B. S., Ogrocki, P., Stout, J. C., Speicher, C. E., and Glaser, R. Marital quality, marital disruption, and immune function. Psychosomatic Medicine 1987, 49:13–33.

26. Kiecolt-Glaser, J. F., Kennedy, S., Malkoff, S. Fisher, L., Spiecher, C. E., and Glaser, R. Marital discord and immunity in males. Psychosomatic Medicine 1988, 50:213–29.

27.   Simonton, C. O., Mathew-Simonton, S., and Creigton, J. Getting Well Again. New York: Bantam Books, , 1980.

28.   Siegel, B. S. Love, Medicine, and Miracles. New York: Harper and Row, 1986.
29.   Newton, B. W. The use of hypnosis in the treatment of cancer patients. American Journal of Clinical Hypnosis 1982-83, 25:104–13.

30.   Grossarth-Maticek, R. Social psychotherapy and course of the disease: First experiences with cancer patients.   Psychotherapy Psychosomatics 1980, 33:129–38.

31.   Bockus, H. L. Gastroenterrlogy., vol. 1.New York: Columbia University Press, 1938.

32.   Alvaraz, W. C. Ways in which emotion can affect the digestive tract. Journal of the American Medical Association 1929, 92:1231–37.

33.   Hartman, H. R. Neurogenic factors in peptic ulcers. Medical Clinics of North America 1933 16:1357.

34.   Jones, F. A. Clinical and social problems of peptic ulcers. British Medical Journal 1957, 1:719–23.

35.   Alexander, F. Emotional factors in gastrointestinal disturbances. In Alexander, F., Psychosomatic Medicine: Its Principles and Application. 1987 NewYork: W. W. Norton.

36.   Mittelmann, B. and Wolff, H. G. Emotions and gastroduodenal function: Experimental studies on patients with gastritis, duodenitis and peptic ulcers. Psychosomatic Medicine 1942, 4:5.

37.   Weiner, H., Thaler, M., Reiser, M., and Mirsky, A. Etiology of duodenal ulcer. I. Relation of specific psychological characteristics to role of gastric secretion (serum pepsinogen). Psychosomatic Medicine 1957, 10(1):1–10.

38.   Alp, M. H., Court, J. H., and Grant, A. K. Personality pattern and emotional stress in the genesis of gastric ulcer. Gut 1970, 11:773–77.

39.   Mirsky, A. Physiologic, psychologic and social determinants in the etiology of duodenal ulcer. American Journal Digestive Disorders 1958, 3:285–314.

40.   Lykestos, G., Arapakis, G., Psaras, M., Photious, I., Blackburn,

I. M. Psychological characteristics of hypertensive and ulcer patients. Journal of Psychosomatic Research 1982, 26(2):255–62.

41. Alexander, F. Emotional factors in cardiovascular disorders. In Alexander, F., Psychosomatic Medicine: Its Principles and Applications. New York: W. W. Norton 1987.

42. Magni, G., DiMario, F., Aggio, L., and Borgherini, G.. Psychosomatic factors and peptic ulcer disease. Hepatogastroenterology 1986, 33(3):131–37.

43. Cattell, R. B. The Scientific Analysis of Personality. Harmondsworth, Middlesex, England: Penguin,1965.

44. Tennant, C. Psychosocial causes of duodenal ulcers. Australian and New Zealand Journal of Psychiatry 1988, 22:195–201.

45. Feldman, M., Walker, P., Green, J. L., and Weingarden, K. Life events, stress, and psychosocial factors in men with peptic ulcer disease: A multidimensional case-controlled study. Gastroenterology 1986, 91(6):1370–79.

46. Walker, P., Luther, J., Samloff, I. M., and Feldman, M. Life events stress and psychosocial factors in men with peptic ulcer disease II. Relationships with serum pepsinogen concentrations and behavioral risk factors. Gastroenterology 1988, 94(2):323–30.

47. U.S. Public Health Services. Reducing the health consequences of smoking: 25 years of progress. A report of the surgeon general. Executive summary, 1989.

48. U.S. Public Health Services. The Health Consequences of Smoking: Cancer and Chronic Lung Disease in the Workplace. A report of the Surgeon General. DHHS publication no. PHS 85-50207. Washington, D.C,.:U.S.Government Printing Office, 1985.

49. U.S. Public Health Service. The Health Consequences of Smoking: Chronic Obstructive Lung Disease. A report of the Surgeon General. DHHS publication no. PHS 84-50205. Washington, D.C.,: U.S. Government Printing Office, 1984.

50. Remington, P. L., Forman, M. R., Gentry, E. M., Marks, J. S., Hogelin, G. C., and Trowbridge, F. L. Current smoking trends in the United States: The 1981–1983 Behavioral Risk Factor Survey. Journal of the American Medical Association 1985, 253:2975–78.

51. Shiffman, S. Relapse following smoking cessation: A situational analyses. Journal of Consulting and Clinical Psychology 1982, 50:71–86.

52. Shiffman, S. A cluster-analytic classification of smoking relapse episodes. Additive Behaviors 1986, 11:295–307.

53. Bare, J. S. and Lichtenstein, E. Classification and prediction of smoking relapse episodes: An exploration of individual differences. Journal of Consulting and Clinical Psychology 1988, 56:104–11.

54. Smith, G. M. Personality and smoking. A review of the empirical literature. In Hunt, W. A. (ed.), Learning Mechanisms and Smoking. Chicago: Aldine, 1970.

55. Spielberger, C. D. and Jacobs, G. A. Personality and smoking behavior. Journal of Personality Assessment 1982, 46:397–403.

56. Eysenck, H. The Causes and Effects of Smoking. London: Temple Smith, 1980.

57. Counsilman, J. J. and MacKay, E. V. Cigarette smoking by pregnant women with particular reference to their past and subsequent breast feeding behavior. Australian and New Zealand Journal of Obstetrics and Gynoecology 1985, 25:101–7.

58. Johnson, E. H. Anger and anxiety as determinants of elevated blood pressure in adolescents: The Tampa Study. Ph.D. dissertation, Department of Psychology, University of South Florida, Tampa, 1984.

59. Johnson, E. H. Emotional and familial determinants of smoking in black and white adolescents. Unpublished manuscript, University of Michigan Medical Center, Ann Arbor, 1989.

60. Gupta, M., Gupta, A., Kirby, S., Weiner, H., Mace, T., Schork, N., Johnson, E. H., Ellis, C., and Voorhees,J. Pruritus in psoriasis: A prospective study of some psychiatric and dermatologic correlates. Archives of Dermatology 1988, 80:1329–34.

61. Gupta, M., Gupta, A., Ellis, C., Kirby, S., Schork, N., Gorr, S., and Voorhees, J. Some psychocutaneous correlates of stress reactivity in psoriasis abstract. Psychosomatic Medicine 1989, 51:254.

5   FIGHTING AND LOVING—SEEING BLACK AND BLUE

1. Luscher, M. The Luscher Color Test. Translated by Ian Scott. Random House: New York, 1969.

2. Straus, M. A. Stress and child abuse. In Kempa, C. H. and Helfer, R. E. (eds.), The Battered Child. 3rd ed., pp. 86–102). Chicago: University of Chicago Press, 1980.

3. Wolfe, D. Child-abusive parents: An empirical review and analysis. Psychological Bulletin 1985, 97(3):462–82.

4. Conger, R. D., McCarty, J. A., Yang, R. K., Lahey, B. B., and Kropp, J. P. Perception of child, child-rearing values, and emotional distress as mediating links between environmental stressors and observed maternal behavior. Child Development 1984, 55:2234–47.

5. Conger, R., Burgess, R., and Barrett, C. Child abuse related to life change and perception of illness: Some preliminary findings. Family Coordinator 1979, 28:73-78.

6. Straus, M.A. . Victims and aggressors in marital violence. American Behavioral Scientist 1980, 23:681–704.

7. Alfaro, J. D. Report on the relationship between child abuse and neglect and later socially deviant behavior. In Hunner, R. J. and Walker, Y. E. (eds.), Exploring the Relationship Between Child Abuse and Delinquency. pp. 175–219. Montclair, N.J.: Allanheld, Osmun, 1981.

8. Spinetta, J. J. and Rigler, D. The child-abusing parent: A psychological review. Psychological Bulletine 1972, 77:296–304.

9. Dodge, K. A., Frame, C. L. Social cognitive biases and deficits in aggressive boys. Child Development 1982, 53:626–35.

10. National Center on Child Abuse and Neglect. Study Findings: National Study of the Incidence and Severity of Child Abuse and Neglect. DHHS publication no. OHDS 81-30329. Washington, D.C.: U.S. Government Printing Office, 1981.

11. Gelles, R. J. and Straus, M. A. Determinants of violence in the family: Toward a theoretical integration. In Burr, W. R., Hill, R., Nye, F. I., and Reiss, J. L. (eds.), Contemporary Theories about the Family. pp. 549–81. New York: Free Press, 1979.

12. American Humane Association, Child Protection Division.

Annual Report, 1980: National Analysis of Official Child Neglect and Abuse Reporting. Denver, Colo.: American Humane Association, 1981.

13. Patterson, G. R. A microsocial analysis of anger and irritable behavior. In Chesney, M. A. and Rosenman, R. H. (eds.), Anger and Hostility in Cardiovascular and Behavioral Disorders, Washington, D.C.: Hemisphere Publishing/McGraw-Hill, 1985.

14. Chamberlain, P. Standardization of a parent report measure. Ph. D. dissertation, University of Oregon, Eugene, 1980.

15. Patterson, G. R. Coercive Family Process. Eugene, Ore.: Castalia, 1982.

16. Reid, J., and Kavanagh, K. A social interactional approach to child abuse: Risk, prevention, and treatment. In Chesney, M. A. and Rosenman, R. H. (eds.), Anger and Hostility in Cardiovascular and Behavioral Disorders, Washington, D.C.: Hemisphere Publishing/McGraw-Hill, 1985.

17. Reid, J. B. Final report: Investigating boys' aggression toward women and girls. Grant R01 MH25548-83, Oregon Social Learning Center, Eugene, 1983.

18. Koneci, V. J. The mediation of aggressive behavior: Arousal level versus anger and cognitive labeling. Journal of Personality and Social Psychology 1975, 32:706–12.

19. Crockenberg, S. Predictors and correlates of anger toward and punitive control of toddlers by adolescent mothers. Child Development 1987, 58:964–75.

20. Engfer, A. and Schneewind, K. A. Causes and consequences of harsh parental punishment. An empirical investigation in a representative sample of 570 German families. Child Abuse and Neglect 1982, 6:129–38.

21. Berkowitz, L. Aversively stimulated aggression: Some parallels and difference in research with animals and humans. American Psychologist 1983, 38:1135–44.

22. Levenson, R. W. and Gottman, J. M. Marital interaction: Physiological linkage and affective exchange. Journal of Personality and Social Psychology 1983, 45:587–97.

23. Julius, M., Harburg, E., and Cottington, E. Marital pair anger-

coping types and all cause mortality in Tecumseh (1971–1983 follow-up). Paper presented at the Gerontological Society of America 39th Annual Scientific Meeting, Chicago, November 19–23, 1986.

24. Tavris, C. Anger: The Misunderstood Emotion. New York: Simon and Schuster, 1982.

25. Johnson, E. H. and Gant, L. Emotional and psychosomatic reactions related to suppressed (anger-in) and expressed (anger-out) anger. Unpublished manuscript, University of Michigan Medical Center, Ann Arbor,1989.

26. Johnson, E. H. The Structured Anger Assessment Interview: Preliminary Manual. Houston, Texas: Behavioral Medicine and Health Psychology Associates, 1990.

27. Frieedman, M. and Rosenman, R. Type-A Behavior and Your Heart. New York: Kropf, 1974.

28. Johnson, E. H. Cardiovascular reactivity during Structured Anger Assessment Interview in black males Psychosomatic Medicine abstract 1989, 51:244.

29. Sherwitz, L., Ross, M., Berton, K., and Leventhal, H. Self-involvement and blood pressure activity in individuals with ischemic heart disease. Unpublished manuscript, 1979.

30. Dimsdale, J. E., Stern, M. J., and Dillon, E. The stress interview as a tool for examining physiological reactivity. Psychosomatic Medicine 1988, 50:64–71.

31. Ebbeson, E., Duncan, B., and Konecni, V. Effects of content of verbal aggression on future verbal aggression: A field experiment. Journal of Experimental Social Psychology 1975, 11:192–204

32. Brown, P. Psychological distress and personal growth among women coping with marital dissolution. Ph.D. dissertation, University of Michigan, Ann Arbor,1976.

33. Brown, P., Perry, L., and Harburg, E. Sex role attitudes and psychological outcome for black and white women experiencing marital dissolution. Journal of Marriage and the Family 1977, August :349–561.

34. Straus, M. A. Wife-beating: How common and why? In Straus, M. A. and Hotaling, G. T. (eds.), The Social Causes of Husband–Wife Violence. Minneapolis: University of Minnesota Press, 1980.

35. Launius, M. and Jensen, B. Interpersonal problem solving skills in battered, counseling, and control women. Journal of Family Violence 1987, 2:151–62.

36. Brehm, S. S. Intimate Relationships. New York: Random House, 1985.

37. Shupe, L. M. Alcohol and crime: A study of the urine alcohol concentration found in 882 persons arrested during or immediately after the commission of a felony. Journal of Criminal Law, Criminology and Police, 1954, 44:661–64.

38. Wolfgang, M. E. and Strohm, R. B. The relationship between alcohol and criminal homicide. Quarterly Journal of Studies on Alcohol 1956, 17:411–25.

39. McKay, J. Problem drinking among juvenile delinquents. Crime and Delinquency 1963, 9:29–38.

40. Selzer, M. L. Alcoholism, mental illness and stress in 96 drivers causing fatal accidents. Behavioral Sciences 1969, 14:1–10.

41. Selzer, M. L,. Payne, C., Westervelt, F., and Quinn, J. Automobile accidents as an expression of psychopathology in an alcoholic population. Quarterly Journal of Studies on Alcohol 1970, 6:34–38.

42. Cameron, N. Personality Development and Psychology: A Dynamic Approach. Boston: Houghton Mifflin, 1963.

43. McMelleand, D. C., Davis, W., Kalin, R., and Wanner, E. The Drinking Man. New York: Free Press, 1972.

44. Tucker, I. F. Adjustment, Models and Mechanisms. New York: Academic Press, 1970.

45. Lang, A. R., Goeckner, D. J., Adesso, V. J., and Marlatt, G. A. Effects of alcohol on aggression in male social drinkers. Journal of Abnormal Psychology 1975, 84:508–18.

46. Borrill, J. A., Rosen, B. K., and Summerfield, A. B. The influence of alcohol on judgement of facial expression of emotion. British Journal of Medical Psychology 1987, 60:71–77.

47. Birhbaum, J. M. , Taylor, T. H., and Parker, E. S. Alcohol and sober mood state in female social drinkers. Alcoholism 1983, 7:362–68.

6   GENDER AND ETHNIC DIFFERENCES IN THE EXPERIENCE AND
    EXPRESSION OF ANGER

1. Maccoby, E. E. and Jacklin, C. N. The Psychology of Sex Differences. Stanford: Stanford University Press, 1974.

2. Hoyenga, K. B. and Hoyenga, K. T. The Question of Sex Differences: Psychological, Cultural, and Biological Issues. Boston: Little, Brown, 1979.

3. Anastasia, A., Cohen, W., and Spatz, D. A. A study of fear and anger in college students through the controlled diary method. Journal of General Psychology 1948, 73:243–48.

4. Sands, D. E. Futher studies on endocrine treatment in adolescence and early adult life. Journal of Mental Science 1954, 100:211–19.

5. Kreuz, L. E. and Rose, R. M. Assessment of aggressive behavior and plasma testosterone in a young criminal population. Psychosomatic Medicine 1972, 34:321–32.

6. Rada, R. T., Laws, D. R., and Kellner, R. Plasma testosterone levels in the rapist. Psychosomatic Medicine 1976, 38:257–68.

7. Scarmella, T. J. and Brown, W. A. Serum testosterone and aggressiveness in hockey players. Psychosomatic Medicine 1978, 40:262–65.

8. Olweus, D., Mattsson, A., Schalling, D., and Low, H. Circulating testosterone levels and aggression in adolescent males: A causal analysis. Psychosomatic Medicine 1988, 50:261–72.

9. Dabbs, J. M., Frady, R. L. Carr, T. S., and Buesch, N. F. Saliva testosterone and criminal violence in young adult prison inmates. Psychosomatic Medicine 1987, 49:174–82.

10. Johnson, E. H. Anger and anxiety as determinants of blood pressure in adolescents: The Tampa Study. Ph.D. dissertation, Department of Psychology, University of South Florida, Tampa, 1984.

11. Johnson, E. H. The role of the experience and expression of

anger and anxiety in elevated blood pressure among black and white adolescents. Journal of the National Medical Association 1989, 81:573–84.

12. Johnson, E. H. The role of anger and anxiety in high blood pressure among black and white adolescents. Advances, 1989, 6:24–27.

13. Johnson, E. H., Kniesley, J., and McManus, J. Psychosocial correlates of perceived distress in adolescents. Adolescence, in press.

14. Siegel, J. M. Anger and cardiovascular risk in adolescents. Health Psychology 1984, 3:293–13.

15. Spielberger, C. D. Professional Manual for theState–Trait Anger Expression Inventory: (STAXI) (research ed.). Tampa, Fla.: Psychological Assessment Resources, 1988.

16. McCann, B. S., Woolfolk, R. L., Lehrer, P. M., Schwarcz, L. Gender differences in the relationship between hostility and the Type A behavior pattern. Journal of Personality Assessment 1987, 51:355–66.

17. Frost, W. D. and Averill, J. R. Sex differences in the everyday experience of anger. Paper presented to the Eastern Psychological Association, Washington, D.C., 1978.

18. Averill, J. R. Anger and Aggression: An Essay on Emotion. New York: Springer-Verlag, 1982.

19. Egerton, M. Passionate women and passionate men: Sex differences in accounting for angry and weeping episodes. British Journal of Social Psychology 1988, 27:51–66.

20. Fitz, D. Anger expression of women and men in five natural locations. Paper presented to the American Psychological Association, New York, 1979.

21. Harburg, E., Blakelock, E. H., and Roeper, P. J. Resentful and reflective coping with arbitrary authority and blood pressure: Detroit. Psychosomatic Medicine 1979, 3:189–202.

22. Frodi, A., Mcaulay, J., and Thome, P. Are women always less aggressive than men? A review of the literature. Psychological Bulletin 1977, 84:634–60.

23. Straus, M. A. Wife-beating: How common and why? In Straus,

M. A. and Hotaling, G. T. (eds.), The Social Causes of Husband–Wife Violence. Minneapolis: University of Minnesota Press, 1980.

24.   Tavaris, C. Anger: The Misunderstood Emotion. New York: Simon and Schuster, 1982.

25.   Rubin, Z., Hill, C. T., Peplau, L. A., and Dunkel-Schetter, C. Self-disclosure in dating couples: Sex roles and the ethic of openness. Journal of Marriage and the Family 1980, 42:305–17.

26. Grier, W. H. and Cobb, P. M. Black Rage. New York: Bantam Books, 1969.

27.   Staples, R. Black Masculinity: The Black Male's Role in American Society. San Francisco: Black Scholar Press, 1982.

28.   Dent, D. J. Readin, ritin, and rage. (How schools are destroying black boys). Essence Magazine, 1989, November:54–59, 116.

29.   Gillum, R. F. Pathophysiology of hypertension in blacks and whites: A review of the basis of racial blood pressure differences. Hypertension 1979, 5:468–75.

30.   Thompson, G. E. Hypertension in black population. Cardiovascular Review and Report 1981, 2:351–57.

31. Clark, K. Dark Ghetto. New York: Harper Torch, 1965.

32. Baughman, E. E. Black Americans. New York: Academic, 1971.

33. Crain, R. L., and Weisman, C. C. Discrimination, Personality, and Achievement: A Survey of Northern Blacks. New York: Seminar, 1972.

34. Yarrow, M. R. (ed.). Interpersonal dynamic in a desegregation process. Journal of Social Issues 1958, 14(1):1–62.

35. Gentry, W. D. Biracial aggression: I. Effect of verbal attack and sex of victim. Journal of Social Psychology 1972, 88:75–82.

36. Fleming, J. and DuBois, L. The Role of Suppressed and Perceived Hostility in Academic Performance: An Exploratory Study of Black Students. New York: Spencer Foundation, 1984.

37. Gentry, W. D. Relationship of anger-coping styles and blood pressure among black Americans. In Chesney, M. A. and Rosenman, R. H. (eds.), Anger and Hostility in Cardiovascular and Behavioral Disorders. Washington, D.C.: HemispherePublishing/McGraw-Hill, 1985.

38. Julius, S. Hemodynamics, pharmacologic and epidemiologic evidence for behavioral factors in human hypertension. In Julius, S. and Bassett, D. R. (eds.), Handbook of Hypertension, vol. 9: Behavioral Factors in Hypertension, Amsterdam: Elsevier Science Publishers, 1987.

39. Esler, M., Julius, S., Zweifler, A,. Randall, O,. Harburg, E., Gardiner, H., and DeQuattro, V. Mild high-renin essential hypertension. Neurogenic human hypertension? New England Journal of Medicine 1977, 296:405–11.

40. Johnson, E. H. Cardiovascular reactivity, emotional factors and home blood pressure in black males with and without a parental history of hypertension. Psychosomatic Medicine 1989, 51:390–403.

41. Dill, B. T. The means to put my child through: Child-rearing goals and strategies among black female servants. In Rogers-Rose, L. F. (ed.), Black Women. Beverly Hills, Calif.: Sage Publications, 1980.

42. Hale, J. E. Black Children: The Roots, Culture, and Learning Styles. Provo, Utah: Brigham Young University Press, 1982.

43. Clynes, M. Generalized Emotion: How it may be produced, and sentic cycle therapy. In Clynes, M. and Panksepp, J. (eds.), Emotions and Psychopathology. New York: Plenum Press, 1988.

7   REGULATING ANGER AND OTHER EXAGGERATED
     EMOTIONAL RESPONSES TO STRESS

1. Ellis, A. How to Live with and without Anger. New York: Reader's Digest Press, 1977.

2. Ellis, A. Techniques of handling anger in marriage. Journal of Marriage and Family Counseling 1976, 2:305–15.

3. Beck, A. T. Depression: Clinical, Experimental and Theoretical Aspects. New York: Harper and Row, 1967.

4. Novaco, R. W. Anger Control: The Development and Evaluation of an Experimental Treatment. Lexington, Mass.: D. C. Heath Lexington Books, 1975.

5. Novaco, R. W. Stress inoculation: A cognitive therapy for anger and its application to the case of depression. Journal of Consulting and Clinical Psychology 1977, 45:600–08.

6. Novaco, R. W. Anger and coping with stress: Cognitive-behavioral interventions. In Forety, J. and Rathjen, D. (eds.), Cognitive Behavior Therapy. New York: Plenum Press, 1978.

7. Wolpe, J. and Lazarus, A. Behavior Therapy Techniques. Oxford, England: Pergamin, 1966.

8. Rimm, D. C., deGroot, J. C., Board, P., Reiman, J., and Dillow, P. V. Systematic desensitization of an anger response. Behavioral Research and Therapy 1971, 9:273–80.

9. Smith, R. E. The use of humor in the counter conditioning of an anger response. Behavior Therapy 1973, 4:576–80.

10. Skinner, B. F. Science and Human Behavior. New York: MacMillian, 1953.

11. Reid, J. B., Patterson, G. R., and Loeber, R. The abused child: Victim, instigator, or innocent bystander. In Bernstein, D. J. (ed.), Response Structure and Organization. Lincoln: University of Nebraska Press, 1982.

12. Patterson, G. R., Chamberlain, P., and Reid, J. B. A comparative evaluation of parent training procedures. Behavior Therapy 1982, 13:638–50.

13. Patterson, G. R. Intervention for boys with conduct problems: Multiple settings, treatments, and criteria. Journal of Consulting and Clinical Psychology 1974, 42:471–81.

14. Patterson, G. R., and Reid, J. B. Intervention for families of aggressive boys: A replication study. Behavior Research and Therapy 1973, 11:1–12.

15. Rimin, D. C., Hill, G. A., Brown, N. H., and Stuart, J. E. Group-assertive training in treatment of expression of inappropriate anger. Psychological Reports 1974, 34:794–98.

16. Pentz, M. A. Assertion training and trainer effects on unassertive and aggressive adolescents. Journal of Counseling Psychology 1980, 27:76–83.

17. Matson, J. and Zeiss, R. Group training of social skills in chronically explosive, severely disturbed psychiatric patients. Behavioral Engineering 1978, 5:41–50.

18. Denicola, J. and Sandler, J. Training abusive parents in child management and self-control skills. Behavior Therapy 1980, 11:263–70.

19. Feindler, E. L and Fremouw WJ. Stress inoculation training for adolescent anger problems. In Meichenbaum N and Jarenko M (Editors), Stress Reduction and Prevention. New York: Plenum, 1983.

20. Roberts, J. and Rowland, M. Vital and health statistics series 11, no. 221: Hypertension in Adults 25–74 Years of Age: United States, 1971–75. DHEW publication no. PHS 81-1671. Washington D. C., Government Printing Office, 1981.

21. Stamler, J., Stamler, R., and Pullman, T. The Epidemiology of Essential Hypertension. New York: Grune and Stratton, 1967.

22. Ward, M. M., Swan, G. E., and Chesney, M. A. Arousal reduction treatment for mild hypertension: a Meta-analysis of recent studies. In Julius, S. and Bassett, D. R. (eds.), Handbook of Hypertension, vol. 9: Behavioral Factors in Hypertension. Amsterdam: Elsevier Science Publications, 1987.

23. Weiss, S. M. Indications for behavioral treatment of hypertension. In Julius, S. and Bassett, D. R. (eds.), Handbook of Hypertension, vol. 9: Behavioral Factors in Hypertension. Amsterdam: Elsevier Science Publications, 1987.

24. Hypertension Detection and Follow-up Program Cooperative Group. Five-year findings of the Hypertension Detection and Follow-up Program. II. Mortality by race, sex, and age. Journal of the American Medical Association 1979, 242:2572–79.

25. Joint National Committee on Detection, Evaluation, and Treatment of High Blood Pressure. The 1984 report of the Joint National Committee on Detection, Evaluation, and Treatment of High Blood Pressure. Archives of Internal Medicine 1984, 144: 1045–57.

26. Weiss, S. M. Stress management in the treatment of hypertension. American Heart Journal 1988, 116:645–49.

27. Johnston, D. W. Psychological intervention in cardiovascular disease. Journal of Psychosomatic Research 1985, 29:447–56.

28. American College of Physicians, Health and Public Policy Committee.Biofeedback for hypertension. Annals of Internal Medicine 1985, 102:709–15.

29. Patel, C., North, and W. R. S. Randomized controlled trial of yoga and biofeedback in the management of hypertension. Lancet 1975, 93–95.

30. Patel, C., Marmot, M. G., and Terry, D. J. Controlled trial of biofeedback-aided behavioral methods in reducing mild hypertension. British Medical Journal 1981, 282:2005–8.

31. Patel, C., and Marmot, M. G. Stress management, blood pressure, and quality of life. Journal of Hypertension 1987, 5(Suppl. 1):S21–S28.

32. Patel C, Marmot MG, Terry DJ, Carruthers M, Hunt B, and Patel M. Trial of relaxation in reducing coronary risk: four-year follow-up. British Medical Journal 1985, 290:1103–06.

33. Patel, C. and Marmot, M. Practice observed: Practice research: Can general practitioners use training in relaxation and management of stress to reduce mild   hypertension? British Medical Journal 1988, 296(6614):21–24.

34. Achmon, J., Granek, M., Golomb, M., and Hart, J. Behavioral treatment of essential hypertension: A comparison between cognitive therapy and biofeedback of heart rate. Psychosomatic Medicine 1989, 51:145–51.

35. Levy, R. L., White, P. D., Stroud, W. D., and Hillman, C. C. Transient tachycardia: Prognostic significane alone and in association with transient hypertension. Journal of the American Medical Association 1945 129:585–88.

36. Paffenbarger, R. S., Jr., Thorne, M. C., and Wing, A. L. Chronic disease in former college students—VIII. Characteristics in youth predisposing to hypertension in later years. American Journal of Epidemiology 1968, 88:25–32.

37. Stamler, J., Berkson, D. M., Dyer, A., Lepper, M. H., Lindberg, H. A., Paul, O., McKean, H., Rhomberg, P., Schoenberger, J. A., Shekelle, R. B., and Stamler, R. Relationship of multiple variables to blood pressure. Findings from four Chicago epidemiologic studies. In Paul O, (ed.) Epidemiology and Control of Hypertension, 307–52. Miami: Symposia Specialists, 1975.

38. Surwit, R. S., Williams, R. B., and Shapiro, D. Behavioral Approaches to Cardiovascular Disorders. New York: Academic Press, 1980.

39. Goldstein, I. B. Biofeedback in the treatment of hypertension. In White, L., Tursky, B. (eds.), Clinical Biofeedback, New York: Guilford Press, 1982.

40. Lee, D., Kimura, S., DeQuattro, V., and Davidson, G. Relaxation therapy blunts pressor response to anger via neutralizing noradrenergic tone. Abstract of the 1989 Annual Meetings of the American Psychosomatic Society. Psychosomatic Medicine, 1989, 51:250.

41. Levenkron, J. D., Cohen, J., Mueller, H., and Fisher, E. Modifying the Type A coronary-prone behavior pattern. Journal of Consulting and Clinical Psychology 1983, 51:192–204.

42. Suinn, R. M. The cardiac stress management program for Type A patients. Cardiac Rehabilitation 1975, 5:13–15.

43. Suinn, R. M., Bloom, L. J. Anxiety management training for Pattern A behavior. Journal of Behavioral Medicine 1978, 11:25–35.
44. Jenni, M. A. and Wollersheim, J. P. Cognitive therapy, stress management training, and the Type A behavior pattern. Cognitive Therapy and Research 1979, 3:61–73.

45. Roskies, E., Spevack, M., Surkis, A., Cohen, G., and Gilman, S. Changing the coronary-prone (Type A) behavior pattern in a nonclinical population. Journal of Behavioral Medicine 1978, 1:201–16.

46. Friedman, M., Thoresen, C. E., Gill, J. J., Ulmer, D., Powell, L,. Thompson, L., Price, V. A., Elek, S. R., Rabin, D. R., Piaget, G., Dixon, T. R., Bourg, E., Levy, R. A., and Tasto, D. L. Feasibility of altering Type A behavior pattern in post-myocardial infarction patients. Circulation 1982, 66:83–92.

47. Freidman, M,. Thoresen, C. E., Gill, J. J,. Powell, L., Ulmer, D., Thompson, L., Price, V. A., Rabin, D. D., Breall, W. S., Dixon, T., Levy, R. A., and Bourg, E. Alteration of Type-A behavior and reduction in cardiac recurrence in post-myocardial infarction patients. American Heart Journal 1984, 108:237–48.

48. Thoresen, C. E., Freidman, M., Powell ,L. H., Gill, J. J., and Ulmer, D. Altering the Type A behavior pattern in postinfarction patients. Journal of Cardiopulmonary Rehabilitation 1985, 5:258–66.

49. Roskies, E. Stress Management for the Healthy Type A: Theory and Practice. New York: Guilford Press, 1987.

50. McLean, E. K. and Tarnopolsky, A. Noise discomfort and mental health. Psychological Medicine 1977, 1:19–62.

51. Knipschild, P. G. Aircraft noise and hypertension. In Tobias, J. V., Jansen, G., and Ward, W. D. (eds.), Noise as a Public Health Problem: Proceedings of the Third International Congress. ASH report no. 10. Rockville, M.D.: American Speech and Hearing Association, 1980.

52. Gradjean, E., Graf, P., Lauber, A., Meier, H. P., and Muller, H. P. A survey of aircraft noise in Switzerland. In Ward, W. D. (ed.), Proceedings of the International Congress on Noise as a Public Health Problem. Washington, D.C.: Government Printing Office, 1973.

53. Paffengarger, R. S., Jr., Hyde, R. T., Wing, A. L., and Hsieh, C. Physical activity, all-cause mortality, and longevity of college alumni. New England Journal of Medicine 1986, 314:605–13.

54. Oberman, A. Exercise and primary prevention of cardiovascular disease. American Journal of Cardiology 1985, 55:10D–20D.

55. Naughton, J. Role of physical activity as a secondary intervention for healthy myocardial infarction. American Journal of Cardiology 1985, 55:21D–26D.

56. deVries, H. A. Tension reduction with exercise. In Margan, W. P. and Goldston, S. E. (eds.), Exercise and Mental Health. Washington, D.C.: Hemisphere Publishing/ McGraw-Hill, 1987.

57. Doyne, E. J., Chambless, D. L., and Beutler, L. E. Aerobic exercise as a treatment for depression in women. Behavior Therapy 1983, 14:434–40.

58. Folkins, C. H. and Sime, W. E. Physical fitness training and mental health. American Psychologist 1981, 36:373–89.

59. Cox, R. H., Hubbard, J. W., Lawler, J. E., Sanders, B. J., and Mitchell, V. P. Exercise training attenuates stress-induced hypertension in the rat. Hypertension 1985, 7:747–51.

Index

child abuse and, 111-12,115-
16, 118;definition of, 47; emotional responses to, 49-52
general adaptation syndrome
and, 44, 47-48; fight/flight
response and, 48-49; management of, 163;physiological
reactions and, 49, 51-52
Structured Anger Assessment
Interview, 120-22; blood pressure response to,120-21, 122

Tampa Study, 60-64; anger
coping in, 61; blood pressure
and, 61-63;smoking, 103-104
Tecumseh Health Study, 28-31,
137
Testosterone, 37; aggression
and, 133-34; violence and, 134
Type-A behavior pattern, 24, 75
alcohol intake and, 80-81;
anger, relation to, 78-80;
cardiovascular reactivity and,
80; components of, 24, 76-77,
79; coronary heart disease
and, 24-25, 77-80; cholesterol

and, 81-82; description of, 24,
76-77; hostility and, 24, 75, 76,
79-80; suppressed anger, 78-
80; treatment for, 165-66

Ulcers, 93-101;anger in, 96-98;
anxiety and, 94, 97-99; de-
dependence and, 94-100
depression and, 97,100; dominance and, 97, 98-99; emotional disturbances and,95, 99-
100; gastric hypersecretion in,
95, 96, 98, 100-01; irritability
and, 98; pepsinogen in, 95-98,
100; peptic, 94, 97, 98, 99-
100; personality characteristics
of, 94, 97-100; psychological
factors in, 96, 99-100; stress
and, 94-95, 98-99; submissiveness and, 96, 97, 98

Western Collaborative Group
Study (WCGS), 77-80
Western Electric Study, 26-27,
35, 37

ABOUT THE AUTHOR

ERNEST H. JOHNSON received his undergraduate and graduate training in psychology at the University of South Florida at Tampa, Florida. His Ph.D. in clinical psychology was granted in 1984. Since that time he has completed specialized training in behavioral medicine and health psychology at the University of Michigan Medical Center where he worked as an Assistant Professor of Internal Medicine until 1989. He also held a position as Associate Professor of Psychology at the University of Houston before recently joining the Department of Psychology and the Behavioral Medicine Research Program at the University of Miami as an Associate Professor. Dr. Johnson has published various articles in professional journals and books on the relationship between personality factors and health.

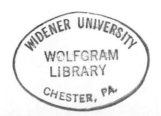